Inspiring Experiences of Arvigo® Practitioners and Their Clients

Journeys in Healing

Compiled and published by the Arvigo Institute, LLC
The Arvigo Techniques of Maya Abdominal Therapy®

Edited by Donna J Zubrod, MSc, MBA, LMBT, CD(DONA),
and Diane MacDonald, RN, MSN, with Rosita Arvigo, DN

Cover Design: Margaret Baker
Interior Design and Page: Jill Shaffer
Copyediting: Nan Fornal

DEDICATION

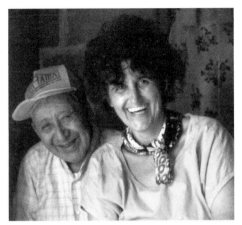

Don Elijio and Rosita, 1990

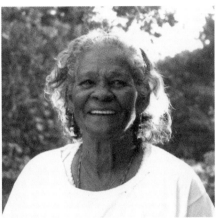

Hortence Robinson, 1928–2009

This compilation of case studies is dedicated to Don Elijio
Panti who passed away in 1996 at the age of 103, and Miss Hortense
Robinson, traditional healer and midwife who passed in November
2009. They were both children of Belizean soil and citizens of
the world. Their lives touched and healed so many with unfailing
generosity, spirituality, humor, and brilliance. To Dr. Rosita Arvigo, DN:
Your contributions to this body of knowledge, known forever as the
Arvigo Techniques of Maya Abdominal Therapy®, will be handed down
through the generations. And to our Arvigo Therapy practitioners, far
and wide across the globe: Your dedication, gifts of healing, and passion
guide us to the future as we heal the world one belly at a time.

ACKNOWLEDGMENTS

Tell me a fact, and I'll learn.
Tell me a truth, and I'll believe.
But tell me a story, and it will
live in my heart forever.
—NATIVE AMERICAN PROVERB

Several years into my therapeutic massage career, I was searching
for something to take my healing practice to the next level. I found
it one morning two years ago on a hilltop in the rainforest of Belize
shortly after Dr. Rosita Arvigo welcomed our Professional Care
Training class on her deck at Villa Rosa. I am very grateful to Rosita
and my instructors, Cathy Lipsky and Megan Assaf, who capably guided
my hands and opened my mind and heart to this work. That week was
life changing; the Arvigo techniques and the expansive community of
like-minded healing professionals fully resonated with me. I jumped in
with both feet and haven't looked back since.

A heartfelt thank you to Rosita Arvigo and the Arvigo Institute
for supporting this project from the beginning; to all the Arvigo
practitioners who provided the compelling stories and the clients that
inspired them; to my treasured husband, Colin Henderson, who has
encouraged me to follow my path and held the home fort many times

so I could readily travel to pursue my Arvigo Therapy studies; to my coeditor Diane and her husband, Steve, for sharing the passionate vision that we could create this book, dedicating many hours, and offering their professional guidance every step of the way; finally to Sam Wise, Tessa, Constance Marie, Jack, Allie, and all the chickens for making me feel at home at the MacDonald homestead in Antrim, New Hampshire, while we worked to bring this book to completion.

—Donna J Zubrod

February 14, 2014

To undertake a project such as this requires dedication, passion, and commitment to promoting the work we do and sharing our successes and challenges as practitioners with one another. This book of client and practitioner experiences began in April 2013 at our practitioner convention in Playa del Carmen, Mexico, and was brought to fruition on the full moon in February 2014. I am forever grateful for the tenacity and driving force given so lovingly by Donna Zubrod, who left hearth and home to spend nearly two weeks in the hills of New Hampshire to bring this to a close. To my dear husband, Steve, who has stood beside me over the years as we worked together to bring the seeds of the Arvigo Therapy into a formal course of study. Thank you to all practitioners far and wide, who are the foundation of our successes, and most of all to Rosita and the traditional healers she learned from. Without this ancient wisdom and knowledge our practitioners would not have the gifts of healing this work has given us. May Arvigo Therapy continue to bring health, healing, and awareness to future generations.

—Diane MacDonald

February 14, 2014

Table of Contents

**Prenatal Wellness, Birth, and
Postnatal Recovery**

CONTENTS

Male Reproductive Conditions

Digestive Disorders and Post-Surgical Recovery

Foreword

Since early childhood, I have been fascinated by the folk cures
of ancient cultures, especially those that address the ailments of women. In
1970 this interest took me to Mexico for seven years, where I met and studied
with traditional healers, midwives, and herbalists. It was a time when modern
medicine had not yet discredited their traditional Mexican home remedies,
massages, and herbal baths. The *curanderas* (healers) and their cures were still
necessary for survival in these remote villages. I remember one blind midwife
in the town of Tlacotepec, Guerrero, who received many of her patients from
hospital referrals. Dark to those who had eyesight, her little one-room clinic
was lined with glass bottles and clay jars full of ointments, salves, and herbs
that she could easily locate by touch or aroma. Like others before her, she had
learned from her grandmother who had learned from her grandmother.

In 1982, after I graduated from the Chicago National College of Naprapathy, my husband Greg (also a naprapath), our young daughter, and I left Chicago in search of medical freedom and land to grow organic food all year. We
packed our worldly goods into a Ford truck to homestead on thirty acres of raw,
uncleared jungle on the Macal River in Cayo District of Western Belize. As
an herbalist and doctor of Naprapathy, it was always my intention to seek out a
teacher in Belize, one who could introduce me to the healing plants of my newly
adopted country. On a hot, sticky afternoon in San Ignacio, I found an old man

sitting on my front porch tapping his black boots on the wooden boards. This visitor was none other than the Maya bush doctor, Don Elijio Panti, of whom I had heard wonderful, wild, and frightful tales. It was a fateful day. The story of my thirteen-year apprenticeship with this old Maya h'men is told in my book *Sastun: My Apprenticeship with a Maya Healer.* During this apprenticeship, I was most impressed with the old master's Maya version of what is known as "folk chiropractic." These are traditional body-work techniques handed down from generation to generation throughout the world's varied cultures.

Don Elijio was internationally famous for his massage for women that centered, lifted, and balanced the uterus. I remember how entire truckloads of women of all ages came to his humble clinic in San Antonio Village to get his *sobada de la matriz,* or uterine massage. Performed with scarred, work-worn hands, his ancient techniques were always gentle, noninvasive, and dramatically effective. For four years I watched this Maya h'men give his massage for women's ailments that ranged from difficult menstruation, lack of menstruation, miscarriages, fertility challenges, uterine fibroids, and ovarian cysts. Don Elijio treated them all with his gentle but deep external pelvic massage, prayers, herbal teas, and vaginal steams. Then, for the next nine years, I gave the treatments under his watchful eye. Don Elijio was an eighty-seven-year-old widower when I met him and one hundred three years old when he passed away in 1996.

As a Doctor of Naprapathy, I am an expert on ligaments of the body. I was immensely impressed with what Don Elijio was able to accomplish with these simple but profound techniques. After ten years of study and research I came to realize that the twelve ligaments that support the uterus in the pelvis respond to strain no differently than do the sixteen ligaments that surround the spinal vertebrae. All ligaments that support body structures can become overstretched or overly taut, a situation that always leads to dis-ease. Poring over books on anatomy, physiology, and medical anthropology for ten years I tried to discern how the old maestro could achieve such astounding results in his humble clinic (in which he treated patients on his own bed in a little eight-by-six cement-block room). I eventually realized that his treatment gently coaxed the uterus into its proper position by massaging the supporting ligaments back to a normal state of tensility so that the body forces of hemodynamics and homeostasis could function undisturbed, unblocked, and unimpeded.

Don Elijio's abdominal massage was also sought after for gastric complaints, which are common in Central America. On average, Don Elijio treated one hundred patients a week. I began recording clients who came to see Don Elijio over a period of seven years. We were able to see that 60 percent of his clients were women with various female complaints; 30 percent were men, women, and children with gastric problems such as lack of appetite, constipation, diarrhea, indigestion, and intestinal gas, and the remaining 10 percent came to see him—the doctor-priest or h'men—for a variety of physical and spiritual problems.

I also had the very good fortune to work with another traditional healer, Miss Hortence Robinson, an herbal midwife of Belize. She was fondly known as *Mil Secretos,* which translates into English as "a thousand secrets." *El Secreto* is a special ingredient—a unique preparation that makes an herbal remedy dramatically effective. This magnificent woman was born in 1928 on Cozumel Island during the days of chicle camps. Her mother and grandmothers were busy midwives there while her father worked the chicle trees. By fascinating coincidence, Cozumel is the ancient home of the Maya Goddess of Medicine, Ix Chel, and the place where the Maya had their school for midwives. Her first teachers were her childhood playmates on Cozumel, the Maya children, with whom she spent a good deal of time collecting medicinal plants for their parents. Delivering her first baby at the age of 13, Miss Hortence delivered thousands more during her lifetime and cared for many sick people who sought her for her simple herbal remedies, massage, and prayers. Although she never learned to read and write, she had an encyclopedic memory and the sharp, retentive mind of a genius. Much of her knowledge was gained by observation and experience of the natural world. She was a living library of knowledge about medicinal plants, home remedies and spiritual healing

I was Miss Hortence's student and friend for more than 25 years and often during that time she was an integral presence at my workshops and talks. Several years ago, Miss Hortence stood proudly by my side before a group of midwives at the Art of Birthing Conference in New York. She received a standing ovation after proclaiming, "I never had a lady tear." I will always remember her love of babies and mothers, and her gentle wisdom and guiding hands. She died in 2009, leaving a legacy of traditional herbal birthing practices in Belize.

Since the early 1990s, with the assistance of many individuals, practitioners, and my students we began to weave the threads of healing that combined Don Elijio's and Miss Hortence's ancient Maya medicine with modern day body-work into what has come to be known as the Arvigo Techniques of Maya Abdominal Therapy®. Through the years, students of varying professions attended workshops and returned with case studies from their practices that demonstrated the benefits of these gentle yet profound techniques. Each class became a learning opportunity as we pieced together the hows and whys of anatomy and physiology for clinical conditions.

Fast forward to the present. We have more than fifteen years of clinical experience from practitioners in varying professions around the world that substantiate the benefits of this therapy. We are committed to preserving the history and lineage of Don Elijio Panti and traditional healers while offering our clients the best of both worlds: time-honored ancient techniques supported by science and easily woven into a practitioner's clinical practice.

Qualified therapists receive a series of seven-day residential trainings that include Self Care Workshops for Maya Abdominal Therapy, Professional Care Training, Pregnancy, Certification, Digestion, and Advanced Clinical Topics. For many years, from 1992 through 2009, I was the only teacher of these workshops. Now, there are dozens of well-trained men and women who have come forward to take over some of the teaching to train practitioners of the Arvigo Techniques of Maya Abdominal Therapy® in twenty countries. Our therapists have backgrounds as medical doctors, acupuncturists, naturopaths, midwives, nurses, nurse practitioners, naprapaths, massage therapists, and chiropractors. Many have contributed their own clinical case histories to this book. Our trainings include the ancient Maya techniques and bodywork that I have personally developed from more than forty years of clinical practice specializing in ailments of women and children. Eventually, Maya Spiritual Healing was added to the training sessions to address the depths of emotional tension so many of us hold in the abdomen.

The case studies in this book show how practitioners of the Arvigo Techniques offered hope when there was none, relief after years of suffering, joy out of despair, and, most of all, they demonstrate how much our self-care massage supports and helps heal our clients. We practitioners work in tandem with our clients, teaching them the gifts of Maya medicine as we look to heal the world one womb, one belly at a time, washing away the tears of inhumanity with each stroke.

—Dr. Rosita Arvigo, DN
San Ignacio, Belize
February 2014

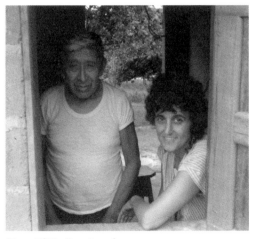

Don Elijio Panti and
Dr. Rosita Arvigo, 1987

A NOTE TO READERS

THE CASE STUDIES presented in this book are actual evidence-based clinical outcomes. The specific Arvigo practitioners have been identified; the client names have been changed to maintain their privacy.

This compilation of case studies reflects Arvigo practitioners' experiences and their practice outcomes. Arvigo practitioners are trained by the Arvigo Institute, LLC, and practice under license or similar legal regulation where they live and work. (Their application of the Arvigo Techniques is governed under that license or regulation, whatever it may be.) The Arvigo Techniques should not be used to diagnose or treat any particular illness or condition or as a replacement or substitute for medical care applied by a qualified medical professional.

The Arvigo Techniques of Maya Abdominal Therapy® may be applied as a complement to medical care, particularly when referred by medical professionals or when seeking symptomatic relief. Additionally, the Arvigo Techniques should not be applied to clients by persons who have not been trained in their use by the Arvigo Institute, LLC, or by persons applying the techniques to self unless instructed in how to do so by a qualified Arvigo practitioner.

Rosita Arvigo, the Arvigo Institute, LLC, and Arvigo practitioners accept no responsibility for use of this book other than as an information resource for examples of how the Arvigo Techniques properly applied by Arvigo practitioners have provided relief and benefit to clients of those practitioners. Therefore, we expressly disavow responsibility for any incidental or consequential damages in connection with, or arising out of, any interpretation or application of the information in this book.

Introduction to Arvigo® Therapy

THE ARVIGO TECHNIQUES OF MAYA ABDOMINAL THERAPY® for the reproductive and digestive systems are external, noninvasive manipulations using only hands to reposition reproductive organs and improve blood flow to digestive organs. Abdominal massage for the reproductive and digestive systems is a therapeutic treatment that has been known and practiced by healers for thousands of years. It was discarded by modern medicine in the twentieth century. Throughout history, healers in Central America have used these techniques in village huts and healing temples. The Arvigo Techniques represent an unbroken chain of knowledge handed down from generation to generation of midwives, healers, and shamans.

These ancient Maya healing techniques eliminate the primary cause of reproductive and digestive complaints in men, women, and children by addressing the congested pelvis and abdomen, thereby preventing the progression of symptoms to chronic disease. The technology that is modern medicine tends to focus on relieving symptoms. Arvigo practitioners are able to apply these techniques to remove the causes of disease.

As is true of the current model of holistic healing, the Arvigo Techniques of Maya Abdominal Therapy® support the body's natural healing capacity. The body's inherent ability to be self-regulating, self-healing, and self-regenerating is known as "homeostasis," or balance within, first recognized by Hippocrates in ancient Greece. As natural healers, we work in the realm of the divine science, removing the obstructions and deterrents to Nature's Healing Force. We do not cure disease. We assist the vital flow of fluids and energy to nourish and repair the organs and systems naturally.

The information presented in the various case studies demonstrates the practitioner's approach to client conditions based on a combination of science and ancient tradition that Dr. Rosita Arvigo has developed over a lifetime. Her years of study in the natural sciences of anatomy, physiology, biochemistry, naprapathy, massage, herbalism, and spiritual healing, as well as more than thirty years of clinical experience, have made it possible to teach practitioners these techniques. Practitioners in turn provide the techniques to their clients.

Women and men suffer needlessly from a barrage of physical complaints that can easily be corrected by returning the uterus and prostate to their proper position and functioning. By applying these techniques practitioners address numerous health issues affecting male and female reproductive systems, digestion, and postsurgical care to name a few. The Arvigo Techniques of Maya Abdominal Therapy® work in partnership with the healing power of nature, or *vix medicatrix naturae*. Paraclesus, a medieval physician, termed this "inherent wisdom."

Those who seek our aid in healing reproductive or digestive complaints already have the elements and mechanisms of healing. However, for any number of reasons they may be blocked because of imbalance in either homeostasis or hemodynamics. Hemodynamics is the study of the dynamics of blood circulation. We have seen what appears miraculous occur within our client's bodies when our hands remove obstacles to the free and dynamic flow of arterial blood carrying nutrients, hormones, and oxygen to the organs.

Homeostasis, defined by Walter Cannon in 1932, is a combination of two Latin words that mean "balance within." It is the property of a living organism to regulate its internal environment to maintain a stable condition by means of adjustments controlled by interrelated regulatory mechanisms. Homeostasis is metabolic equilibrium maintained by complex biological mechanisms that operate via the autonomic nervous system to offset disruptive changes. Through homeostasis our bodies are able to adapt themselves to fluctuating conditions within and without.

Female Reproductive Issues and Fertility Enhancement

Healing from a Lifetime of Painful Periods

*The uterus is the woman's core.
If it is out of balance, her
whole life is out of balance—
physically, emotionally, mentally
and spiritually.*

—DON ELIJIO PANTI

Madeleine As I write this I am 30 years old. I realize now that for
most of my life I have been disconnected from my reproductive cycle
and my sexuality. I was on the birth control pill from when I was about
17 until I was 26. During this time I experienced several relationships
and sexual encounters that left me feeling hollow and unlovable. For
me, sexual connection became divorced from emotional connection.
At one point, when I was 26, I had an unwanted sexual experience that
left me feeling full of shame, fear, and distrust.

When I was 27 I switched to a copper IUD (intrauterine device)
for birth control. My menstrual cycle was starting to be regulated by
my own hormones, and my body was starting to adjust back to its
natural state. Around this time I started getting back in touch with my
body and emotions and I fell in love with a man that I later married.
I don't have much recollection of what my periods were like before
I had the IUD, but the longer I had the IUD, the more pain I was
experiencing. My menstrual cramps during the first one to two days
of bleeding were very uncomfortable. What really did me in, however,

was the pain that arrived a week after my period. Somehow I knew it was not normal menstrual pain—it always started a few days after my period had ended, and the pain was different. It made me feel cold and nauseated. I felt a stabbing in my lower abdomen. Ibuprofen sometimes took the edge off but never helped much. On the worst days, I found relief only by going to bed with a hot water bottle, waiting for the pain to pass. Apparently I had bacterial vaginosis that was unrelenting. Further medical tests revealed no obvious cause and the doctors all told me that I had dysmennorhea and that the IUD was not the reason for my intense pain and chronic vaginal infection.

My situation remained the same for another two years. All the while I continued to explore methods to eliminate the pain and discomfort. I had acupuncture regularly. I learned about herbs that support the female reproductive system and began drinking a quart of herbal tea daily. I took nutritional supplements, used homeopathy, and tried any remedy for bacterial vaginosis that I could find. I explored, researched, and experimented, yet the pain and nausea intensified.

The day that I finally got the IUD removed is blazed in my memory. As soon as the IUD was out of my body, I felt waves of warmth rush to my lower abdomen. I felt euphoric. I felt vindicated. The nurse practitioner who removed the IUD told me that one of the arms was bent, probably had gotten bent during insertion, and could have been poking me in the uterus that whole time. The non-period pain immediately went away as did the bacterial vaginosis. My first menstrual cycle without the IUD washed away the dried blood that had been accumulating inside my body for more than two years.

From then on, I have come to know and trust my body even more. I have had the support to continue the work of integrating my emotions and sexuality. I have been learning how to be kinder to myself. I still typically have fairly strong cramps on the first two days of my menstrual cycle. When the cramping is at its worst, it is accompanied by nausea and diarrhea, and I can barely stand upright. The hot water bottle and bed rest are the only things that offer me comfort. These intense period cramps are what led me to enroll in a Self-Care Workshop to learn more about the Arvigo Techniques of Maya Abdominal Therapy®. I had read somewhere on the Internet that these techniques might help me with my painful periods.

PRACTITIONER PERSPECTIVE   The first Arvigo Therapy session that Madeleine received was the 20-minute anterior abdominal massage that is included in the Self-Care class I taught during May 2013. I have the students in the class fill out the full Arvigo medical history intake form for their own benefit of self-reflection, for the benefit of the Arvigo practitioner performing the mini session, and also to use in the future as a gauge of what has changed since starting the abdominal self-care massage or using the other tools taught in the Self-Care class.

Madeleine's abdominal muscles felt tight during the mini session, with the uterus feeling low and full since it was close to her menses, so the lower abdominal massage strokes were done lightly. The upper abdomen also felt tight and from reading her intake form and discussing her past sexual history, I sensed this was emotional armoring. Energetically, my impression from the session was that Madeleine's abdomen has been a place where past hurts have been stored and that it would take time for these emotions to clear for her. My style of treatment with the massage is to proceed energetically at where the person is at and not push into where the tissue is not ready to release. I felt that personal self care would be Madeleine's best route for self healing, both in her womb and in her heart energy.

I was very impressed by Madeleine's resolve to incorporate healing activities into her life, as well as daily self-care massage and taking Female Tonic herbal tincture. Her desire to incorporate activities that are both beautiful, connected to nature, and grounding will provide a good foundation for her physical, emotional, and spiritual healing.

Over the next several summer months, I saw Madeleine twice in my acupuncture clinic around week 4 of her cycle. My treatment plan has been to open, move, and soothe the energy around her lower abdomen.

At the end of that summer, Madeleine came to see me to receive her first full Arvigo Therapy session. She reported to me at that time that her period symptoms were improving. However, she was experiencing some consistent right sciatic leg pain that ran laterally from her sacrum down the back of her leg. Compared to when I first worked with Madeleine, the tissues of her abdomen were about 50 percent softer and more mobile. Her uterus was slightly low but had improved mobility. I sensed tightness and lymph congestion—a feeling of resistance against my pressure—in Madeleine's left lower abdomen and around her navel. When I assessed her posterior, I noted that her pelvic bones were misaligned. Madeleine's right mid back and gluteal area (the side of her sciatic pain and the side of where one of the arms of the copper IUD had been irritating her uterus) showed visible signs of tissue congestion. I corrected her pelvic alignment and continued with the posterior Arvigo Therapy treatment. At the end of her session, Madeleine reported she felt very good and relaxed and that the sciatic pain had lessened.

My role is to continue to support Madeleine in her healing journey—a journey that as one can see from her story has its ups and downs. In the long run, however, Madeleine is experiencing significant benefits from her self-care efforts.

Madeleine's Experience

Since the May Self-Care workshop, I have had several menstrual cycles. My first period came in June just 4 days after the workshop, and my cramps were still pretty bad. They were not as bad as previously, however, because I began menstruating at night and the cramps did not wake me as they usually did. During my next cycle I implemented several self-care activities: I planted an herb garden in early June; I made myself a little home altar which I tend to daily with fresh cut flowers and stand before and ground myself in the morning, I consistently did the self-care massage 3 to 5 times a week and took Female Tonic herbal tincture 10 to 14 days before menstruation, and I started consistently receiving acupuncture in week 3 or 4 of my cycle. I learned that my adrenal glands were fatigued, and I started taking supplements for that. I also suspected that I was gluten intolerant and began a gluten-free diet to see if I would notice any changes in my symptoms. The next time my period came in July I still had cramps, but they were nowhere near as debilitating as usual! The pain was much less and I had almost no diarrhea or nausea. This was a huge change for me.

When August came along, I could barely stand when my period came on. It was painful and exhausting. My husband had just left for California the day before, where he would be for 4 months. I had been less consistent with the abdominal self-care massage in the preceding weeks, and had been feeling a lot of anxiety and sadness about his impending departure. It hit me hard when he left, and I guess it hit me in the uterus, too.

Now it is September, and I am glad to report that this month has again been an easier one, with only moderate cramps and no diarrhea or nausea. I still miss my husband a ton, but the initial gut-wrenching impact seems to have worn off. I am in the stage of maintaining now, and figuring out what I need to do for myself to stay balanced in the next few months. I am continuing to do things that nourish me, such as pottery classes and seeing my therapist. I'm being consistent with my self-care massage and taking the Female Tonic. I went to a weekend meditation retreat at the beginning of the month that really reached me. I now meditate every morning for 10 minutes at my home altar. According to my doctor, my adrenal function is starting to improve.

In many ways, I am grateful to my cramps. They have motivated me to explore and really learn what it means to care for myself. I am also grateful to Li-Lan for her support and for introducing me to the Arvigo Techniques of Maya Abdominal Therapy®. She helped me to understand the importance of taking care of myself and inspired me to take a self-care journey and embrace the things that nurture and heal me most.

I am curious to see what my future cycles will bring!

 Li-Lan Hsiang Weiss LaC (www.armoniahealth.com) Li-Lan, licensed acupuncturist, has been incorporating the Arvigo Techniques of Maya Abdominal Therapy® into her Oriental medicine practice since 2008. She is a certified Arvigo instructor for both the one-day Hands on Health the Maya Way workshop and the transformative Self-Care class. Dr. Rosita Arvigo's teachings have had a significant impact on Li-Lan's reconnection to the beauty, sacredness, mystery, and healing power within our bodies and in nature. She helps clients rediscover and understand their innate healing capacity through the poetic language of Chinese medicine and the embodiment practices of the Arvigo techniques. Li-Lan's practice focuses on reproductive, digestive, and emotional well-being for women, men, and children; she is fluent in Spanish and Mandarin.

Dysmenorrhea   Pain associated with menstruation, dysmenorrhea, is the most commonly reported menstrual disorder. More than half of women who menstruate have pain 1 to 2 days a month. There are two types of dysmenorrhea. Primary dysmenorrhea relates to muscle cramping as the uterus is shedding its lining, and it ends with the period. Secondary is caused by a disorder in the reproductive system (endometriosis, adhesions, fibroids), and pain can be felt anytime during the menstrual cycle. Recent research incorporating Doppler radar confirms that women with primary dysmenorrhea experience pain due to low blood flow to their uteri both during their periods and also at all times throughout their menstrual cycles. Typical treatments for dysmenorrhea include hormonal medications such as birth control pills, antiinflammatory drugs, and insertion of an IUD. For the more severe cases, surgery is recommended, with hysterectomy as a last resort.

Finally! Relief from Painful and Irregular Periods

*Healing yourself is connected
with healing others.*

—YOKO ONO

Hannah The first time I got my period in my early teens I had to stay home as I was incapacitated with nausea and vomiting from the severe menstrual cramps. Every month thereafter I experienced similar unrelenting pain. I was very active athletically with gymnastics, softball, volleyball, tennis, skiing, and cheerleading so when that time of month came I was unable to participate fully in my activities, if at all.

When I was 22, it was recommended that I go on the birth control pill to help manage the pain. However, the accompanying side effects for me were so severe that I took the pill for only 6 weeks as I experienced chest pain, nausea, vomiting, breakthrough bleeding, swelling of my lip and fingers. I was crushed. There was no reprieve from the dreadful discomfort. My cycle was very irregular and came anywhere from 24 to 32 days and 5 to 7 days, with super heavy flow and clotting for 3 to 4 of those days. I also noticed that one month I would have cervical fluid and the other month I wouldn't. This irregularity with my cervical fluid made me think that I wasn't ovulating regularly.

I studied to become a registered nurse, specializing in intensive care and trauma, eventually becoming a perfusionist (a specialist who operates a heart-lung machine during open-heart surgery). By the time I reached my 30s I had pain all the time on the left side of my lower abdomen and not just when I menstruated. My job was very demanding, and many times I had to ask a coworker to assist me at work because the cramping, nausea, and sporadic vomiting were so severe.

One afternoon, at the age of 38, I was jumping rope in the driveway, when all of a sudden I wet my pants, with urine running down my legs. This was very emotional for me since I did not know what was going on. Sobbing, I asked myself, "Am I that old that I am starting to become incontinent?" I felt very depressed, and I couldn't stop crying. The next day my period arrived and stayed for 19 days. My appointment with my ob/gyn revealed my hormones were out of balance and my uterus was tipped, but that there was nothing that could be done aside from surgery to clip the uterine ligaments and put the uterus back into place. I did not want to have surgery and felt there must be another way. I found myself wanting to leap off the table and run away. An ultrasound was scheduled, which revealed a cyst on the left ovary about the size of three cherries.

Interestingly, a friend of mine told me she was at a dinner engagement and met two interesting people from Belize, Dr. Rosita Arvigo and her husband, Greg Shropshire. She suggested I read a book by Dr. Arvigo, *Sastun,* which recounted her apprenticeship with a Maya shaman. After I read this book, I immediately knew in my heart that Dr. Arvigo could help me in some way. I contacted her in Belize and she let me know when her next Self-Care Training class on the Arvigo Techniques of Maya Abdominal Therapy® was scheduled. I registered immediately and was excited about my upcoming class.

PRACTITIONER PERSPECTIVE   Hannah contacted me and attended my very next scheduled Arvigo Self-Care Training workshop. During the class I worked on her and noted her uterus was indeed malpositioned and was lying low and toward the left in her abdomen. From her signs and symptoms I felt there was a possibility that her uterus could be anteflexed (bent over forward on itself). I explained to Hannah it was abnormal to have such painful periods and that by applying these self-care techniques she could manually assist her uterus to shift to a balanced, supported position, which would allow it to function more effectively. I recommended that she be diligent with performing her self-care massage daily; even twice a day would be beneficial. She should also wear a faja after she did her self-care to help support her uterus's proper position until the ligaments were strong enough to support the uterus on their own. She was advised to be patient as natural healing doesn't happen immediately, but most likely she would start seeing improvement with her next cycle.

Hannah's Experience Doing the self-care massage was wonderful! It felt so good that I did it twice a day, and it helped to alleviate the left side discomfort almost immediately. Within a month my pain had diminished significantly and I felt it was easier for my uterus to stay in place with the support of the faja, which I wore under my hospital scrubs. By the 2-month mark I had regular cycles with cervical mucus, 5 healthy days of bleeding without urinary stress incontinence, no nausea, and almost no pain. I continued with the faja for 3.5 months after starting self-care massage as wearing it felt very supportive while I was working.

A couple of months after I started the self-care massage, an intravaginal ultrasound was repeated to evaluate the status of the ovarian cyst. During this procedure I performed some of the self-care technique and the technicians saw my uterus move. They were shocked at how I was able to lift and move my uterus with this simple massage. One of them commented, "No one's uterus is in the right place; everyone's is low or tipped. We see it all the time." To which I replied, "Just because you see it all the time doesn't mean it's supposed to be that way." The good news was that the cyst on my ovary was reduced in size by 75 percent.

I was committed to continuing my self-care massage daily because it made my body feel good. After 7 months I could honestly say that I was consistently having no abdominal pain for the first time in my life.

At this time I had a follow-up annual wellness appointment with my ob/gyn. He was surprised with my results. Aside from his comment about how well I looked in general, my tests showed that my hormones were balanced and my physical exam showed adequate cervical fluid and a uterus in proper position. He asked me what I did to improve my results and I told him about the Arvigo Techniques of Maya Abdominal Therapy® and the accompanying daily self-care techniques. He replied, "Well, there are things that aren't in the medical books that work. Good for you." I made a commitment to myself that I would continue self-care massage for another year and then planned to decide whether or not I would pursue professional training in the Arvigo Techniques of Maya Abdominal Therapy®.

Over the next year I realized this work had been transformative, allowing me to nurture myself and become more connected to my feminine nature. Through my nursing career I have come to realize that Western medicine doesn't always have the answers. I admired the holistic approach of Arvigo Therapy and how it empowers people to help them heal themselves and evolve. I decided to work toward becoming a certified practitioner and teacher of the Arvigo Techniques of Maya Abdominal Therapy®.

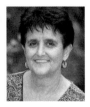 **Rosita Arvigo** DN   Dr. Rosita Arvigo is a naprapathic physician, herbalist, international lecturer, and author. She has lived in Central America for more than 30 years and has studied with various traditional healers, the most notable of whom was Don Elijio Panti, the renowned Maya shaman of Belize. She is the author of *Sastun: My Apprentice with a Maya Healer,* and coauthor of *Rainforest Remedies: 100 Healing Herbs of Belize, Rainforest Home Remedies: How to Nourish Your Soul the Maya Way,* and *The Art of Spiritual Bathing.* Dr. Arvigo directs the Ix Chel Tropical Research Foundation in Belize, is a founding member of the Traditional Healers Foundation, and operates the Ix Chel Wellness Center in Santa Elena, Belize. She was awarded the Wings Trust Women of Discovery Earth Award for 2003.

An Integrated Treatment Approach for for Chronic Debilitating Menstrual Pain

Learning to form mutually
nurturing relationships,
as part of a commitment to love
and nurture ourselves on every
level, will improve the health of
every organ in the body.

—CHRISTIANE NORTHRUP, MD

Attia My periods were never easy, beginning with the painful first day and ending to a lesser extent on the fourth day. Along with the pain, I would bleed heavily the first two days and had poor digestion. I was still able to function, but by the summer of 2011 the cramps were worsening with less menstrual flow. Most of the time during my period I would stay in bed trying to find comfort. I was 27 years old at the time without any surgical history, pregnancies, or trauma.

My turning point happened in September of that year as I was getting ready to drive from Maine to Indiana to start a new job. Just before I was scheduled to leave, I started my period, experiencing an unprecedented amount of pain and being able to do little else than sit on the floor with a heating pad, staring blankly at music videos. My rear and legs felt like they had taken a beating. A friend applied massage to these areas and this eventually offered me some relief. Four days later I was on the road to Indiana!

My pain centered in the lower abdomen just above the bladder where (I thought!) my uterus was, and in my lower back with the worst being in the pelvic floor. This was a change from past years where the pain was more in the lower abdomen. A massage therapist I was working with described it well for me. It was as if I was "giving birth to demons."

I knew something wasn't right and sought the services of a nurse practitioner who worked with allopathic and herbal approaches. A hormone test revealed I was very estrogen dominant for my age, and she started me on a natural progesterone cream that I was to apply to my wrists during the second part of my cycle. Fall arrived, but the progesterone was not helping at all. The menstrual pain was spreading out to days before and after menses, requiring me to miss a day or two of work each month at my brand-new job. Oral contraception was recommended, and I tried a low estrogen product that did not make a difference.

At this point my nurse practitioner ordered an ultrasound, which showed a normal, arcuate uterus (a variation in which the uterine fundus displays a concave contour toward the uterine cavity). Next was a consult with an ob/gyn, who suggested Lupron if I was willing to take it as it would stop my periods and shrink the endometrial implants if that was indeed the source of my pain.

In April of 2012 a laparoscopy was done to confirm if endometriosis was present. The laparoscopy only took about an hour and showed no signs of endometriosis, only adhesions connecting the bowel to the left side of my body and a slightly dilated bowel. The pain during recovery was not too bad. However, my cycle that started a week following the surgery was the worst pain ever and required me to stay home for another week. A few weeks after the surgery, I began a series of seven weekly pelvic floor therapy sessions. The physical therapist felt that the main issue was muscle tightness, difficulty releasing the tension. By performing Kegel exercises and manual stretches of the vaginal walls, along with other exercises and an electrode stimulation machine, I found some relief.

Online research led me to the "endometriosis diet," which excluded inflammatory and estrogenic foods: wheat/gluten, dairy, red meat, alcohol, unfermented soy, and sugar. I adopted this diet full time with the exception of completely eliminating sugar. My digestive symptoms improved; I lost weight and was able to take pain medications when the cramps were severe. In addition to dietary changes, I began yoga, started acupuncture treatments, and continued pain medications but had a feeling they did not reach the core of the problem.

I began a new relationship, but intimacy was infrequent for many reasons including my frequent cycles. When we did engage in intercourse, it was quite painful for me. I remember one time when after a few short minutes of intercourse (which felt good, during), I had to place an ice pack on my vulva.

At this point the difficult decision was made; I decided to stop my periods and began the first of 3 monthly Lupron injections in August of 2012. I felt released from the fear of the next month of horrific pain, but started having very low energy and became more depressed as the symptoms of menopause set in. Other stressors in my life added to a decrease in confidence as well. Even when on Lupron, I could feel the constant pressure in my pelvic floor, as if something was being pinched. I had the feeling that when my periods came back, the terrible pain would too.

My acupuncturist referred me to Megan Assaf, who was a practitioner of the Arvigo Techniques of Maya Abdominal Therapy®. I had my first visit with her early in October 2012. She felt my uterus was malpositioned and began applying the techniques. During the session I felt something inside move and shift up and forward. The best description I can share is that it felt like a set of internal suspenders had been pulled up and within a few hours the lingering pain was gone.

PRACTITIONER PERSPECTIVE   In October of 2012 I saw Attia for her first Arvigo Therapy session. She presented with a history of chronic debilitating menstrual pain that often left her on the floor. I was struck with how much this pain had interfered with her life including her sex life. In the last year she had been prescribed a variety of medications to manage her hormones and the pain, but none of them were helping her. Exploratory surgery to look for the cause of the pain was inconclusive. I was impressed with the way she was not willing to accept her status quo: She continued to seek out treatment options including physical therapy and other self-help techniques such as changing her diet.

My initial determination was that her uterus was malpositioned and, given her symptoms, most likely retroverted (leaning against the descending colon). The tissue in her lower abdomen felt puffy, inflamed, and tender. After applying the abdominal massage it was apparent that the tension was decreased and I felt less congestion toward the back of her abdomen. Along the way, Attia experienced different sensations in her body as her pelvis shifted, which are common signs of the flows of blood, lymph, nerve, and energy starting to move through the area again, as well as balanced pelvis and ligament structures. We discussed a uterine-friendly lifestyle, including self-care aspects that were particular to decreasing inflammation.

She returned for her second session two months later, reporting her menses was still painful yet tolerable. Arvigo Therapy was applied, and it was evident there were changes in her status from the previous session. I sensed that her uterus was not as posterior but to the left side of her pelvic bowl. Once again, I gently massaged and balanced the pelvis.

We worked together until April 2013, at which time I referred her to work with a second Arvigo practitioner because of scheduling challenges. She continued to make progress from May to August as her symptoms slowly improved and her home self care was consistent.

At the time of this writing, it has been nearly a year since Attia's initial therapy session with me. Her symptoms have improved significantly since the days when she would lie on the floor in excruciating pain. With time I anticipate Attia's situation to improve even more, as the inflammation from chronic congestion continues to clear, her uterine ligaments continue to strengthen, and she works on her pelvic floor strength and continues to be committed to her self-care massage and lifestyle habits.

Attias' Experience

Working with Megan has taught me that there is no magic bullet to overcoming menstrual pain from a malpositioned uterus, but that it is a step-by-step process in which the patient herself must be a full participant.

After my initial session with Megan I began menstruating again within a month. While still painful, my next period was bearable. Learning self-care massage was an important component to add to my routine. I continued with my monthly Arvigo Therapy sessions, performing self-care massage, and following an anti-inflammatory diet and uterus-supportive lifestyle. The body awareness I was developing during this time was very interesting. For example, I flew to Wisconsin in March 2013 for a job interview, and I was so delighted that my unexpected period didn't ruin the interview! On the return flight home I had to lift my heavy carry-on bag to the overhead compartment. As I lifted it overhead, I felt my uterus drop. The rest of the period became moderately painful and the blood flow lighter, which I surmise was due to my uterine position suddenly changing. This reinforced for me that my self-care habits need to be an ongoing priority for me.

To further enhance my awareness I enrolled in an Arvigo Self-Care class Megan was teaching. As part of this two-and-a-half-day class I participated in a meditation that consciously connected with the energy and spirit of my uterus. During the meditation, my uterus told me that I had treated her as a liability instead of an asset over the past years. We engaged in a meditative dialogue, where I promised not to work against her again and to continue with the self-care massage. I feel the message I received at this time aided in my healing.

In early July 2013 I had a repeat transvaginal ultrasound while performing self-care massage. To my surprise my uterus was in an anteverted position, with each stroke resulting in a retroverted movement. It was amazing to see at the end of each stroke how the uterus floated up again.

While my improvement has been gradual, the extreme symptoms are gone. I am no longer on birth control or other medication during menses. Pain is manageable with castor oil packs, vaginal steams, and decreasing life stressors. For me, healing is a matter of learning new habits that are supportive to me.

It is now September 2013 and during this cycle I had a period that was better than any I have had over the past two years. I actually went hiking on the second day, something that would have been unthinkable even six months ago! I think that I am at the point where I no longer need to receive regular monthly Arvigo Therapy sessions as my self-care massage and lifestyle habits are working for me. Arvigo Therapy and my Arvigo practitioners not only have given me a set of tools, but they have also given me hope and inner strength. With healing as with life in general, many have helped me, but, ultimately, the one responsible for my success is me.

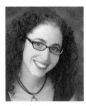 **Megan Assaf** BFA, CMT, C-MAT (www.wombsforwisdom.com) Megan has been in private practice since 2000, offering detailed and intuitive massage therapies. She specializes in chronic pain relief, women's care, and energy and abdominal therapies. A passionate educator, she has taught both nationally and internationally for the Arvigo Institute at the Self Care and Professional Intern levels. She is the artisan and developer of Wombs for Wisdom anatomical uterine models.

Managing the Pain of Endometriosis

The mind will use the muscles and organs of the body as an outlet for pent up emotions.

—WILHELM REICH

Kelly I have been diagnosed with endometriosis, and for years suffered with daily pelvic pain that radiates down my legs and up to my lower back. No amount of pain medication relieves this pain. Living in pain every day is frustrating and exhausting and affects every area of my life. Often at work the pain is so severe I lie on the floor writhing in distress. In addition, emotionally I am moody and tired, and intercourse is painful, which affects my relationship. I can easily say this has led to a low quality of life.

Megan Assaf was teaching a one-hour introductory presentation on the Arvigo Techniques of Maya Abdominal Therapy® at Cleansing Waters that I had RSVPed to attend. This particular Friday evening I was tired, weak, and hungry but went anyway as something deep inside me was calling me to go. I felt this would be important information for my healing journey, so I headed over despite my physical and emotional state. I am grateful that I showed up because I was completely blown away by Megan's presentation. A deep knowing seeped through my whole body while I listened to her talk about Arvigo Therapy. I knew without a doubt that I would work with Megan.

PRACTITIONER PERSPECTIVE   I saw Kelly as a client after she had heard me speak about Arvigo therapy and how it could help women with endometriosis. She presented with extreme pain that was typically every month and not limited to just her menstrual time, occasionally happening before menses or also around ovulation. Kelly had already altered her diet to be endometriosis-friendly, being a wonderful advocate for herself and a great researcher, and having arrived to see me with a set of self-help skills already happening.

In working with clients with this condition, it is important to address as best we can the numerous causes of this condition. One theory is retrograde menstruation (menstrual blood backflows into the fallopian tubes, enters circulation); a malpositioned womb is another potential cause as are dietary issues. Our first priority in working together was to bring the womb into optimal position and alignment. The second goal was to decrease inflammation through the use of castor oil packs and dietary and other lifestyle changes. Vaginal steams (bajos) would be used to assist in the cleansing of hard and fibrous tissue on the uterine wall. Most important would be client patience and persistence to assist and support the body to heal.

Kelly's initial session included my assessment and treatment with the focus on her lower pelvic bowl. During this session, she spontaneously experienced an emotional response to the treatment, which is not uncommon and often assists the healing process. Following this experience, she was glowing, radiant, and more present in her body awareness. We continued to work together over the next few months to help her body to shift until she was confident to take over her own care.

Kelly was dedicated to using the tools we discussed, and with each session we saw incremental progress, with less and less pain and difficulty, until she was ready to go down to a maintenance level in her therapy, which is now four times a year. Occasionally, Kelly's symptoms will flare up as the endometriosis responds to environmental or lifestyle factors, but Kelly reports managing those times skillfully and is able to navigate through them well with her self-care tools. Kelly is a prime example of how faith, persistence, and being committed to self-care day by day can result in more health and vitality.

Kelly's experience

My first session with Megan was an amazing experience. During the first hour, Megan placed a heated castor oil pack on my abdomen, and I lay on the table while we went over my medical history. I received the Arvigo Therapy during the second hour of my session. As Megan massaged my abdomen, I felt as though an avalanche of stored emotions was pouring out of me. I cried and screamed as the emotions were purging. I began to feel light as Megan continued to gently massage my womb. I felt pressure and a pulling sensation, feeling my uterus begin to move. When the session was complete, I no longer felt pressure or pinching in the pelvic area, feeling my uterus was now upright. When I walked out of Megan's office, I was walking differently than ever before. My steps were light, and my eyes were clear . . . all the way to my soul.

Integral to the Arvigo Therapy is self care. I continue to apply castor oil packs on myself at home, I've changed my diet and lifestyle, and I do the self-care massage. I may not do the self-care massage every day, but I do it regularly enough to notice a difference. I continue to see Megan four times a year for a professional Arvigo Therapy session.

My greatest benefit from this work for the last two years is that I am no longer living in pain. My menstrual cycles are manageable now. I no longer experience daily pelvic pain. If I need pain relief during my cycle, then one Advil is enough to ease the pain. Sex is no longer painful, and the pain in my legs is now gone. My mood is stable, and I have a significantly greater quality of life.

Megan Assaf's professional biography appears on page 36.

Endometriosis When tissue that forms the lining of the uterus (endometrium) is found outside of the uterus in the abdominal cavity, the diagnosis is endometriosis. It occurs in about 10 percent of women of reproductive age and is most often diagnosed when they're in their 30s and 40s. The places where the escaping endometrial tissue ends up are called implants, and they're usually found on the peritoneum, ovaries, fallopian tubes, outer surface of the uterus, bladder, ureters, intestines, rectum, and behind the uterus. Endometrial tissue responds to changes in estrogen level, so the implants grow and bleed like the uterine lining does during the menstrual cycle, causing surrounding tissue to become inflamed, irritated, and swollen. Eventually, the implants form scar tissue/adhesions, causing organs to stick together. Pain comes from cyclic implant bleeding, inflammation, and scar tissue, especially before and during menstruation. This process can result in chronic, long-term pelvic pain, pain during sex, pain based on where the implants are located (if implants are on rectum, for example, then there could be pain during bowel movements; if implants are on the bladder, there could be pain while urinating). It is interesting that many women with endometriosis have no symptoms. Almost 40 percent of women with infertility have endometriosis as resulting inflammation can damage sperm or egg and interfere with movement through the fallopian tubes. In severe cases, fallopian tubes can be blocked by adhesions. The only way to confirm endometriosis is by laparoscopy. The condition is treated with anti-inflammatory and hormonal medications. Surgery to remove the endometriosis and adhesions is also an option. After surgery most women experience pain relief. However, 40 to 80 percent will have pain again within 2 years as surgery is not a cure for endometriosis. Hysterectomy is a last-resort surgical option.

Diligence with Self Care Addresses Frequent Urinary Tract Infections

Everything in the universe is within you. Ask all from yourself.

—RUMI

Nora I am a 32-year-old high school history teacher, track coach, and avid runner. Since I was in college I have experienced four to five urinary tract infections per year. I've had numerous studies to find out if there were other causes for my frequent infections such as kidney stones, bladder spasms or a bladder without tone, sexually transmitted diseases, or diabetes, and thankfully was free of these conditions.

I am a single woman, presently not in a long-term relationship. I do not smoke or take any medications. I enjoy running about 30 miles a week as it relieves my stress and provides me with a sense that all is right with the world. The only problem I experience with running is painful "stitches" beneath my ribs if I don't concentrate on my breathing.

Overall, my health is good, so I could not understand why I continued to get frequent urinary tract infections. My menstrual cycles had some cramping at the beginning not associated with the infections. The infections were not associated with seasonal changes. I changed my diet to avoid processed foods, flour, and sugar. This helped for a short time but not significantly.

A colleague, also a runner, told me about a self-care massage she was taught by a nurse practitioner who specializes in the Arvigo Techniques of Maya Abdominal Therapy®. The colleague had gone to her because she was having trouble holding her urine while running and wound up wearing a cloth belt wrap to keep her uterus in place while she ran. She mentioned that she does her self-care massage almost every day and and no longer has a problem with holding her urine.

After another infection, I finally decided to call the nurse practitioner, Cathy Lipsky, and made an appointment. I was surprised at the amount of time she took with me; our session was interactive and informative. Cathy asked me the most unusual questions such as what kind of underwear I wore and if I ever felt heavy "down there." Once she finished with the questions, she explained everything that she would be doing and taught me how to do a self-care massage for myself. I felt so taken care of and supported.

PRACTITIONER PERSPECTIVE   I first saw Nora shortly after treatment she had for a urinary tract infection and at the end of her menstrual cycle. Reviewing her menstrual history, I saw that she had irregular blood flow and noticeable heaviness and bloating in her pelvic area prior to her period. She reported that testing was done to rule out any pathology that might cause the urinary tract infections, and all tests returned normal.

Some forms of underwear and sanitary products can predispose women to urinary tract infections, so prior to getting Nora on the treatment table, I asked her what kind of underwear she wore, and she reported that she usually wears thongs except when she has her period and that she uses tampons on occasion.

Evaluating Nora's lower abdomen, I found that her uterus was low and anterior. Her upper abdomen showed a tight band just beneath her breastbone extending below both sets of ribs with tension down the midline of her abdomen. I suspected that the tension in her upper abdomen could be causing her "stitches" while running. Continuing the evaluation, I found her pelvic bones were misaligned and her low back muscles were tight and tender upon palpation. She also had significant tension around her sacrum.

During the session she noticed a "buzzing sensation," which I explained was due to increased circulation and energy moving through her body while at the same time releasing chemicals much like the endorphins that are released during running. Prior to the end of her session, we spent time reviewing the instructions for her self-care massage, wearing a faja (a supportive cloth belt) when running, not to wear thongs for at least a month, and if she had to use tampons, to try organic unbleached cotton. Nora was troubled about not wearing thongs, but I explained that the thong portion of the underwear (just like the string from the tampon) can slide back and forth between the anal area and the vagina and urethra contaminating both orifices and becoming a vehicle for infection. She agreed to accept my suggestions, and we made a second appointment for her to return prior to her next menses.

A few days after the session, I followed up with Nora and she reported she was enjoying her new self-care routine, but reported having a dark mucus discharge that she recalled from our discussion may be a normal response to her uterus cleansing itself, which I reinforced for her. In addition, she was pleased to see how her body was responding to self care and felt the faja was providing support when running.

At our second visit Nora reported that after two weeks she noticed changes in her own pelvic area as well as her upper abdomen, feeling these areas were softer. She was pleased with the changes and felt she was connecting with her body. In applying the Arvigo Therapy, I confirmed the soft areas she found in her lower abdomen and pelvic bowl and explained this was due to increased circulation. Nora's ability to support herself in her healing quest was very apparent.

At our third session a few weeks later, Nora reported additional changes: The heaviness in her pelvis near her menses was gone, her flow was regular, and, most intriguing, the "stitches" were gone when she ran. Over her next few cycles we continued to work together. The changes included a gradual reduction in tension in her lower pelvis; her menstrual flow continued to regulate. Most important, however, was four months went by without a urinary tract infection since our first session! She continues to run with the faja, uses tampons only when absolutely necessary, and wears thong underwear only on occasion.

Nora's Experience

It's been 18 months since I started working with Cathy and during this time I have had only minimal symptoms of a potential urinary tract infection for which I took some herbs but did not need medical treatment. I remain diligent with doing my self-care massage, and I continue to see Cathy on a monthly basis around the middle of my cycle.

I have been blown away at my journey into self healing because of my experience with Arvigo Therapy. Never in my wildest dreams would I have thought that the position of my uterus could be the reason for my many urinary tract infections. Now I know that if I feel a sensation, I can increase the amount of times I do my self-care massage and begin taking herbs to cleanse my urinary tract. I now feel connected to my cycle and uterus and blessed to be reconnected with my feminine nature. I am more aware of my body, and I can appreciate how it can restore itself with my help.

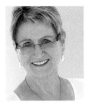

Cathy Lipsky RN, NP (www.holisticnp.com)   Cathy Lipsky is a nurse practitioner with more than 40 years of experience taking care of the adult population. Since 1997 she has learned from her mentor, Rosita Arvigo, how valuable self care is as part of a healing practice and has used the Arvigo Techniques of Maya Abdominal Therapy® in her practice of holistic therapies in New York. A certified practitioner as well as a Self Care and Professional level teacher of the Arvigo Therapies, Cathy continues her studies with Rosita in order to support and continue the healing work that the ancient teachings have provided. Cathy has served as a member of the Advisory Board of the Arvigo Institute and sits on many committees, reviewing and revising the current trainings and guidelines that the Arvigo Institute has created over the years.

Urinary Tract Infections   Also known as acute cystitis or bladder infection, a urinary tract infection (UTI) can cause painful, burning urination, frequent or intense urges to urinate even when there is little urine to pass, back pain, and cloudy, dark, bloody or foul-smelling urine. A UTI can begin anywhere along the urinary tract, which includes the urethra, bladder, and kidneys. A UTI occurs when one or more of these organs become infected, usually by the bacteria *Escherichia coli (E. coli)* that live in the bowel.

People of any age or sex can get UTIs; however women are four times more likely than men to get them, with UTIs being most prevalent among young, sexually active women. Women have a shorter urethra, which makes it easier for bacteria to reach the bladder; the opening of a woman's urethra is near the vagina and anus, where bacteria live. Half of women will have at least one infection at some point in their lives. Recurrences are common; 20 percent of women who have had a UTI will experience another, and some women have three or more UTIs a year. Lifestyle changes may help prevent repeat UTIs. Even though the symptoms are daunting, most UTIs are not serious. In uncomplicated cases, urinary tract infections are easily treated with a short course of antibiotics, although resistance to many of the antibiotics used to treat UTIs is increasing. In complicated cases, longer course or intravenous antibiotics may be needed, and if symptoms have not improved in two or three days, further diagnostic testing is necessary as these infections can lead to serious problems if left untreated.

Challenging Fibroids

The female pelvis is a powerhouse of energy transformation.

—DR. ROSITA ARVIGO

Catherine I heard about Maya Uterine Massage from a friend who attended an introductory talk given by Diane MacDonald. It was the fall of 1998, and no one I knew had ever heard of this type of treatment. My husband and I had been married for a short time and wanted to start a family. However, my fibroids were causing me a problem in conceiving. I was 18 when diagnosed with uterine fibroids; most of the small ones were at the top of the uterus and in the walls, but the one of major concern was a large one (apple-sized) sitting near the opening of my cervix and leaning on my bladder. No one had been able to tell me how or why I developed fibroids at such an early age, other than my mother had them when she was in her 30s. My doctor was a specialist in uro-gynecology and had been seeing me on a regular basis for 10 years since the fibroids appeared. I looked at every health care option, from surgery to natural approaches and had done everything known at that time. My diet was organic, vegetarian; I took special enzymes, decreased stress, everything! After my friend told me about the uterine massage, it piqued my interest as it was an option other than surgery.

PRACTITIONER PERSPECTIVE Catherine called me for information to address her fibroids. I had just completed my Professional Care Training and was the only practitioner in New Hampshire at that time qualified to practice Maya Uterine Massage (as it was known back then). I knew working with clients with fibroids could be challenging due to size, location, and lifestyle issues, to name a few. We had a lengthy phone discussion about her situation and scheduled her first session. Catherine was hopeful this treatment along with everything else she was doing would shrink the fibroids, especially the larger one, so she would be able to conceive.

At our first session I noted her uterus was enlarged to just below the navel with a firm bulging area at her pubis to about an inch above. It was easy to palpate the uterine edges and feel some of the fibroids externally. A castor oil pack was applied before and after the session, which included a full anterior and posterior treatment. She was instructed in self-care massage, home castor oil packs, and vaginal steams. We discussed the use of Female Tonic, but she was already taking herbal remedies from an acupuncturist she was working with.

Catherine and I continued to work together two to three times a month as her schedule allowed since a visit to my office necessitated 90 minutes' travel one way! She was compliant with the home routine and started to feel changes with her uterus. Over the next 6 months I observed her uterus begin to get smaller at the navel, slowly decreasing to about 2 inches above the pubic bone. The edges of the uterine wall were smoother, and tissue in the pelvic bowl was palpable and soft. However, the fullness at her pubic bone did not change.

My recommendation was for Catherine to have another ultrasound to determine if the therapy was making a difference as we had been working together for 6 months. It turned out that she was scheduled for a repeat ultrasound at her annual visit with her surgeon. The ultrasound showed that the smaller fibroids at the top (fundus) and wall of the uterus were not present, but the larger one was still the same.

Catherine's experience

The sessions with Diane were really amazing. She gently massaged my womb while I would visualize each cell of my fibroids to melt. Home self care was a pleasure to do as it gave me something else to focus on. My husband and I were hopeful that we would indeed be able to conceive. The follow-up ultrasound was reassuring to be sure, but the surgeon was concerned about the larger fibroid at the base of the uterus near the cervix. We discussed surgical options again. I saw Diane for a few more sessions before surgery. The plan was to remove the fibroid or have a hysterectomy as the surgeon wasn't sure how easy the surgery was going to be. These sessions were focused on preparation for surgery, knowing that the outcome could go either way.

A month after surgery I saw Diane one last time. As it turned out, I had a hysterectomy. The fibroid at the base of the uterus was bulging out of the uterine wall and adhering to the bladder. According to my doctor, it would have been only a matter of time before the fibroid invaded the bladder. Even though my husband I and made this decision, I feel the work Diane and I did supported me to say goodbye to my womb. Interestingly, I felt free after the surgery as my energy was no longer focused on dealing with fibroids. My home self-care and uterine massage sessions eliminated the smaller ones, which was reassuring. About 2 months after surgery I began applying the self-care massage to decrease post-surgical adhesions from forming. It was a gentle way for me to stay in contact with the soul of my womb that was no longer present. We are planning to adopt children in the future and know this is the best decision for us!

PRACTITIONER NOTE   This early case study and other practitioner experiences in working with fibroids soon became the foundation of the Arvigo Therapy fibroid protocol, *which gives hope and guidance to practitioners and clients they work with.* Fibroids are a challenging condition to address. However, in combination with conventional medicine, Arvigo Therapy offers an alternative option for treatment as well as support if other procedures are indicated.

 Diane MacDonald RN, MSN   Diane MacDonald is the program administrator and certified instructor for the Arvigo Institute, LLC. Working in nursing since 1982 in numerous medical settings as an RN, manager, and family nurse practitioner, she presently maintains her private practice in Antrim, New Hampshire, working with a variety of client populations with Arvigo Therapy, health and wellness, and stress reduction. She has worked in developing the Arvigo Institute, LLC, and its core content since 2001. Diane is one of the first teachers to complete an internship with Dr. Arvigo, in 2000, to teach Professional Care classes. She has assisted Dr. Arvigo in all of the workshops and since 2001 has taught classes in the US and internationally in the UK, Australia, and Israel.

Fibroids   Benign growths that develop from the muscle tissue of the uterus are called uterine fibroids. The size, shape, and location of fibroids can vary greatly; inside the uterus, on its outer surface, within its wall, or attached by a stem-like structure. Fibroids are fairly common and occur in up to 80 percent of all women by the time they're 50. Fibroids may cause symptoms (menstrual changes, pressure, pain, enlarged abdomen, infertility, miscarriages), but most of the time fibroids do not cause symptoms, and a woman is usually unaware of their presence. She may develop one or many of varying sizes and locations. A fibroid may remain small for a long time and suddenly grow rapidly, or grow slowly over a number of years. The cause of fibroids is unknown; genetic and vascular system abnormalities and tissue response to injury have been suggested as playing a role in their development. There is often a history of fibroids developing in women of the same family. Women of African descent are two to three times more likely to develop fibroids than women of other races. Fibroid growth depends on estrogen, which is why it is rare for them to develop until after puberty. Fibroids are most common in women aged 30 to 40. Uterine fibroids tend to shrink or disappear after menopause, when estrogen levels fall. If symptoms become serious, treatment may include pain or hormone medications, or a hormone releasing IUD. More serious fibroids may require surgery. A myomectomy removes the fibroid, leaving the uterus intact; a hysterectomy is a last resort if the fibroid is very large and other treatments are unsuccessful.

A Game Change for Living with Vaginal Prolapse and Urinary Incontinence

We are what we repeatedly do.
Excellence, therefore, is not
an act but a habit.

—ARISTOTLE

Ruth I am an elderly, postmenopausal woman and have been dealing with bladder control for more than 15 years, initially starting with slight urine leakage. About ten years ago I participated in a research trial that a local teaching hospital was conducting where I learned some pelvic floor exercises, including Kegel exercises. They helped minimize my bladder control issues, but only for a while. I have used panty liners for more than a decade, slowly graduating to heavier protection and now use them about 80 percent of the time.

Two years ago I felt something bulging from my vagina; doctors determined this protrusion was my vaginal wall. Following several visits to doctors and undergoing a variety of tests, it seemed a pessary was the best option for me. After the pessary was inserted, I had no bladder control for a week. I asked for the pessary to be removed, feeling I would have to live with the prolapse, but it continued to be a problem. I have a part-time job that I enjoy, and I am very active for my age. I couldn't stand or sit for long without feeling my vaginal wall start to slip out. I also noticed that my urinary incontinence was getting worse, and as my bladder filled I would experience disturbing pressure and pain. My quality of life was suffering. I wanted to keep my part-time job and continue my active life. However, I was concerned that if my situation continued to worsen I would become completely housebound.

Several months later a dear friend told me about the Arvigo Techniques of Maya Abdominal Therapy® and how it had helped her with urinary incontinence. I decided to find out more about this therapy. I felt fortunate when I learned there was an Arvigo Therapy practitioner, Donna Zubrod, who practiced just ten minutes from my home in North Carolina.

At my initial session, Donna showed me how to perform some simple massage techniques on my abdomen and also explained how the Arvigo Therapy would help to improve my condition. I consistently performed my daily abdominal self-care massage routine. It took only ten minutes, and I found it easy to remember to do it nightly at bedtime.

PRACTITIONER PERSPECTIVE When I first met Ruth, I was struck by her determination to improve her condition. The urinary incontinence and vaginal prolapse had taken a toll on her. Standing upright led to her vaginal wall protruding which was a nuisance and very uncomfortable. She felt the pelvic floor exercises she did to help alleviate her symptoms were no longer helping. All her symptoms were gradually becoming worse.

As I worked with Ruth, both her upper and lower abdomen were extremely sensitive to touch, and her tissues underneath my hands were immobile. Her uterus was positioned low and anterior. Her pelvic bones were imbalanced; both hips were tilted anteriorly, and her right hip was elevated more than her left. The tissues above her sacrum felt puffy and appeared swollen, telling me there was a circulation issue, and her sacrum lacked mobility.

Ruth was relaxed during and after her Arvigo Therapy session. She actually slept as I was treating her. I recommended a regimen of daily abdominal self-care massage with a pillow under her hips to elevate her pelvis and to continue her pelvic floor exercises. Ruth was somewhat dehydrated from avoiding drinking water to minimize urinating to avoid leakage, so I encouraged her to do her best to increase her water intake to help with her healing.

Ruth contacted me the next day, having experienced significant leg discomfort overnight and was also feeling lightheaded. I explained to her that Arvigo Therapy was helping to increase circulation throughout her abdomen bringing fresh blood and nutrients to tissues and organs and that they likely had not been receiving fresh blood and nutrients for quite some time. I continued to explain that this natural healing process was likely causing some new and unusual symptoms for her, but that this would be temporary. Ruth called me the next day to let me know that her new symptoms were gone.

Two weeks later she returned for her second session, reporting some positive results. The urinary leakage was less, and she felt she was able to empty her bladder more completely when urinating. In addition, she felt the vaginal protrusion was less. When she manually repositioned it into her body, it would stay in place longer when she was standing. This allowed her to feel much more comfortable standing on her feet and working for longer periods of time. Her pelvic muscles felt stronger, and she also felt that while she was doing her exercises they were more productive.

At this visit, I noted that her upper and lower abdominal tissues were less sensitive to touch and were more mobile, allowing me to work at deeper tissue levels. Her uterus was no longer low and anterior, but more neutral and upright with a sense of movement to it. Ruth's sacrum still looked a bit swollen and felt puffy and immobile, but her pelvic bones were more balanced than before.

Ruth returned for her third session nearly two months later. She had a big smile on her face when she told me that since her initial visit, she had missed only two days of doing her self-care massage. Clearly, her diligence paid off in wellness benefits. Ruth beamed as she reported that she could now stand for an entire day without her vaginal wall protruding, and when it did happen, it was minimal. During the day she had no urinary incontinence. When I assessed her, I found that her uterus position was still neutral, and all her abdominal tissues and organs had good mobility. Her pelvis was still continuing to rebalance itself. Her sacrum no longer appeared swollen, and I was finally able to feel it move. Ruth had experienced many positive changes in her condition in less than three months!

I now work with Ruth once every three months for maintenance. She remains faithful and committed to her self-care massage and pelvic floor exercises. Over the past year her symptoms have diminished significantly, and what remains she feels she can easily manage. For the first time in 15 years, Ruth no longer has to restrict her activities or lifestyle.

Ruth's Experience

My symptoms started to change for the better within the first week after my initial session with Donna. After two months of daily self-care massage and two additional Arvigo Therapy sessions, I'm delighted with how my condition has improved! I have few issues of leaking urine as my bladder control and vaginal muscles feel stronger. I only feel the protrusion after standing or walking 30 minutes or more and it no longer causes discomfort while I'm seated or lying down. There is no sense of disturbing pressure and pain as my bladder fills, and gone are the adult diapers; medium absorbency pads are adequate if I need them. When I do my physical therapy exercises to help strengthen my pelvic floor, the activity feels more productive. I can actually feel the muscles I am supposed to be working, whereas before I had very little sensation down there while doing the exercises. My pelvic floor feels stronger and more supportive now. I am committed to daily self-care massage and exercises to help my condition continue to improve. Thank you, Arvigo Therapy, for giving me my life back.

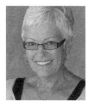

Donna J Zubrod MSc, MBA, LMBT, CD(DONA) (www.sevengenerationswellness.com) Donna is a nationally certified, North Carolina licensed massage and bodywork therapist, and birth doula. Her practice, Seven Generations Massage & Birth, supports women toward positive experiences and outcomes during their childbearing years through menopause and beyond. As a certified Arvigo Therapy practitioner with advanced women's wellness training, she has helped couples with fertility challenges to successfully conceive, nurtured expectant mothers during pregnancy through postpartum, and offered relief to clients from discomforts caused by stressful or active lifestyles, women's wellness issues, traumatic accidents, and surgeries.

Navigating Perimenopause

*Where is the one who will open
their heart to this hard work?*

—DON ELIJIO PANTI

Angela   I'm 42 now, and I started my periods around the age of 13. They have always been heavy and a problem, but in the last few years they have become intolerable. I have been back to my doctor on numerous occasions, complaining about pain, heavy bleeding, depression, mood swings, problems sleeping, vaginal dryness, cystitis-like symptoms, including blood in my urine, and a whole host of other problems.

Eventually, my doctor tested me and said my hormone levels suggested I was perimenopausal. He offered me pills to help me sleep, pills to help with my moods, and not a lot else. I was becoming desperate. My moods affected the whole family—my husband, 9-year-old son, and 14-year-old daughter. I love my husband very much, and he has been endlessly supportive, but some days I could barely get out of bed to do more than the absolutely necessary.

The pain would start with ovulation, which some months could be crippling, and then the mood would slowly descend into darkness. The first few days after I finish bleeding are the best each month, but that is in fact a small window of only a week or so. The pain, the exhaustion, and the depression were ruining my life, so when Hilary Lewin offered me a series of Arvigo Therapy treatments and I understood how they might help me and my symptoms, I jumped at the chance.

PRACTITIONER PERSPECTIVE   Angela came to me in a state of despair. She felt written off by her doctor, and her only hope was that at some point she would reach menopause and she would leave the pain and depression behind. Her menstrual cycles had never been easy, and whilst she valued herself as a woman, she felt let down by her womb.

Her first session with me was very moving; she shared her story of sexual trauma as a teenager and the loss of her father in the fourth month of her second pregnancy. We talked about how these emotions can be held in our bodies and the power of nurturing herself each day with the self-care massage.

The first session I applied the Arvigo Therapy techniques with a feather-light touch on her abdomen and equally gentle on her back. She shed a few tears, seemed to enjoy the session, and was keen to return for more treatments.

I saw her three more times at 2-week intervals, and her progress was a joy to watch unfold. The tightness in her belly fell away, and she was able to tolerate deeper work. The sacrum which had initially felt puffy and congested improved, and the colour of her skin changed from a blue tinge to pink over the weeks that we worked together.

Angela was able to find time each day to do the self-care massage, and this has become an important part of her life.

Angela's Experience
During my first Arvigo Therapy treatment with Hilary, I experienced strange spasms in my belly. I was not asleep, but it was though I dreamt of my teenage self and I said goodbye to her. I had never completely let go of her; I still feel her, but it felt good to let her go. The next day I started my period. It was several days early but it was amazing as I had no pain!

After my next session I had no breast tenderness. I am sleeping better and generally feeling less anxious and tired. I love doing the self-care massage as it feels really positive.

The most amazing thing is that I then had no pain on ovulation which has historically been worse than my periods. You have no idea how good it feels to be coping with life again, and my husband and kids are starting to notice a difference.

This work has taught me a way of listening to my body and somehow seems to have alleviated so many of those symptoms my doctor had no answer for. The bladder symptoms are slowly improving; there is no more blood in my urine, and I am confident I will continue to improve.

A combination of being listened to, having a clearer understanding about what is going on each month with my body, and learning some new ways to look after myself has been life changing. I am bringing my daughter to see Hilary soon as I think so much of this should be taught to teenage girls in school. If we as women understood our bodies better, we would be able to explain ourselves more clearly and access better treatment. Arvigo Therapy should be available to all women at least once in their lives.

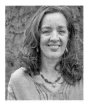 Hilary Lewin (www.suistherapies.co.uk) Hilary has joyfully been spreading the Arvigo "word" around the planet for some years after discovering the work, studying it in the States, and bringing it back to the UK. As a massage therapist and founder of Doula UK, Hilary found that the Arvigo Techniques of Maya Abdominal Therapy® filled in the missing gaps. She has trained as an Arvigo instructor and now teaches therapists around the world. She practices from Guildford, Surrey, working with women and men at all stages of life and has developed a reputation as a straight-talking therapist who helps people to help themselves. Hilary is currently working on a post-natal programme to support women through the first 40 days after birth.

Stored Emotions and Trauma: Resolving Issues in Your Tissues

*The failure to restore
homeostasis is at the basis for
the maladaptive and debilitating
symptoms of trauma.*

—PETER A. LEVINE

Marla   I have experienced two miscarriages in the last three years. I was so excited when I found out that I was pregnant the first time that I let everyone know as soon as I found out. When I miscarried, it was so hard for me to tell my family and friends. I felt ashamed and exposed and that I was letting everyone down; this would have been the first grandchild on either side of the family. When we conceived the second time, I was determined to wait to tell everyone the good news until I was further along in the pregnancy and out of miscarriage danger. Unfortunately, my second miscarriage came at 16 weeks, later in my pregnancy than the first, so it was fairly complicated. I ended up having to have a D&C procedure to complete the miscarriage, and I found this quite traumatic. I still had not told my family or friends about my second pregnancy, so when this trauma happened I had only my husband to lean on for support. He did what he could but was fairly traumatized himself and was limited in the support he could provide me.

My follow-up exam with my ob/gyn was very uncomfortable. During my pelvic exam the doctor casually mentioned that I had a retroverted uterus. I had no clue what this meant or if it could be impacting me in any way. I looked it up online and read in a post that something called the Arvigo Techniques of Maya Abdominal Therapy® could influence uterine position. When I checked the Arvigo Therapy website I found an Arvigo practitioner, Mickey Sperlich, who practiced not far from my home.

PRACTITIONER PERSPECTIVE   Marla is a 28-year-old woman who contacted me about "infertility issues." She had read that Arvigo Therapy might be able to help and was eager to, as she said, "try anything." While going through her health history with her, I learned that Marla was not actually currently trying to conceive; she had experienced two miscarriages and was not actively trying to get pregnant. Marla also shared with me that she had had several significant falls as a young girl and teenager, that her periods had always been pretty rough for her, and that she had some discomfort at the time of ovulation. On her session intake form she put a question mark for the response to the question about any history of abuse, and she indicated that she was currently feeling depressed. When we discussed her responses, she did not elaborate on her "question mark" response and I did not press her for any details. I did share my beliefs about how emotions get stored in the body—that I am aware of this and professionally trained to walk through this with her as I do with all my clients.

During her session Marla shed a few gentle tears and expressed some momentary discomfort which prompted us to take a couple of breaks. On the whole, however, she was receptive to the treatment and commented on areas of tension she was experiencing by saying things like, "Wow, I didn't know I was so tense there." She did seem to have a lot of core belly tension, some sacral torsion, and some pelvic misalignment. I also confirmed the uterine finding of retroversion. I treated these findings and showed Marla how to do the self-care massage and recommended she take Female Tonic to address her painful and profuse menses and painful ovulation.

At Marla's second session a month later she began right away with sharing what she experienced since she last saw me. While she was performing her self-care massage, Marla said she had memories of pediatrician visits when she was quite a little girl that she had always thought were normal but which she had remembered were always extremely uncomfortable. She remembered being told to undress and being digitally examined by the doctor on more than one occasion. She also remembered how scared and alone she felt when this happened as her mother was outside in the waiting room. Her self-care massage also made her think a lot about her traumatic second miscarriage, and she said she felt her pediatrician visits and miscarriage were linked in some way. Marla asked me directly what I thought about that. I validated for her that these experiences did seem quite similar; that she seemed to have felt both trauma and helplessness in both situations; and that she also felt that she was all alone during both these times in her life. Although I did not name this trauma for her as rape, I did validate her feelings and suggest to her that it might be worthwhile for her to talk to a mental health professional to explore this further. She said she would think about it. I performed the Arvigo Therapy session and noted an improvement in her uterine position and her pelvic alignment. Marla also reported that her menses pain and flow were showing signs of getting better. I recommended she continue with her daily self-care massage and Female Tonic.

When Marla came to see me a month later, she discussed her trauma memories even more. This time she seemed to want my opinion about what she was remembering. Did I think it was abuse? I told her that she was the expert on that. Regardless of whether there was a legitimate reason for the digital exams by the pediatrician, her experience of them was indeed traumatic and worthy of further exploration. I reiterated my recommendation of seeing a professional to guide her and referred her to a trauma-informed mental health practitioner, whom she agreed to see.

Arvigo Therapy can help clients to work toward resolution of past traumas and grief. While addressing the abdominal healing that is the central focus of our work, the therapy can reveal how the physical and emotional are intertwined and how all components need to be addressed for complete healing.

Marla's Experience

My cycles are getting easier for me. The self-care massage feels very good, but I am overwhelmed by my thoughts and memories that have been coming up for me while I'm doing it. I have shared details of these disturbing memories with Mickey, and I am questioning what they are all about. Mickey has been a supportive listener during our sessions together, and I am grateful for having her validate my feelings. I have so many unanswered questions and confused feelings about what I am remembering, and whether they are impacting my ability to carry a baby, that I have decided to follow up on Mickey's recommendation to see a mental health practitioner that she has referred other clients to and who specializes in working with people dealing with trauma. I need help with dealing and resolving these memories from my childhood and the grief of my miscarriages before I can move forward with having children of my own.

PRACTITIONER NOTE   So as to assure client confidentiality, Marla's case study is a composite of several of my clients, each with a history of sexual trauma.

I am a retired midwife, a researcher, a doctoral student, and Arvigo Therapy practitioner. My area of research is looking at the way that a history of sexual and other interpersonal trauma exposure affects childbearing processes. Because of this, I bring a trauma-informed lens to my work with my clients. While I maintain primary focus on the needs and concerns that clients bring with them into sessions, I also inquire about trauma exposures; not only whether they have had the falls and abdominal surgeries that we typically associate with uterine displacement, but also whether they have experienced sexual trauma, including rape, incest, or other abuse, and whether they have ever entered into treatment for any mental health challenges related to such exposure. Many women are resilient in their recovery from trauma and do not have enduring mental health problems. However, I have found that regardless of the positive adaptations we may make psychologically to deal with insults to our beings, nonetheless, the body remembers—and such trauma often leaves resonance, in our bellies, specifically.

Childhood sexual abuse in the US is distressingly common, with estimates ranging from 10 percent to 51 percent, depending on the population studied. In preparing this contribution, the researcher in me wanted to verify these statistics in my own client data. Toward that end I looked at my files for the last 100 clients I have served.

In my practice 48 percent of my clients reported a significant physical trauma of some kind; 37 percent reported a history of sexual trauma specifically; and 14 percent reported both types of exposures. Only 29 percent of clients reported no significant trauma. It is beyond the scope of practice for Arvigo Therapy practitioners to perform formal mental health assessment. However, inquiring into a client's history is important, relevant, and within the scope of practice. In my practice, 18 percent of the last 100 clients I have served endorsed current depression. Although these percentages in the US and in my practice are already high, there is reason to believe that these numbers are a conservative estimate of the true rate of trauma exposure when you take into consideration that many women are choosing not to share this information with their practitioners, and that many women may have dissociated from their trauma to the degree that they are unable to recall their trauma in a complete way.

Addressing trauma as a health care or bodywork professional should be axiomatic; we should be normalizing this experience in that we provide opportunities for disclosure (or nondisclosure), stand ready to listen, show empathy, provide respectful and appropriate treatment, and adapt our care as necessary, and stand ready with referrals to mental health practitioners for trauma-specific mental health treatment. It is important for me to be open and honest with my clients about the potential for emotional exploration to occur and how it may open doors to further healing. In my work with clients it appears that we judge ourselves for having such emotions when they emerge.

I commend Dr. Rosita Arvigo for ensuring this aspect of the work is a central component of the training for practitioners. We as practitioners can listen to, support, and refer to mental health professionals who can further work at addressing these issues.

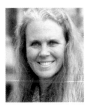 **Mickey Sperlich** MA, MSW, CPM (mickeys@wayne.edu) Mickey retired from a long and fulfilling midwifery career several years ago in order to pursue her interest in research on the effects of trauma on the lives of childbearing women. Her first research project resulted in the award-winning book, *Survivor Moms: Women's Stories of Birthing, Mothering, and Healing.* She worked for several years on a research team at the University of Michigan in Ann Arbor, investigating the effects of trauma and posttraumatic stress during pregnancy and the postpartum period. She is currently finishing a doctoral degree in social work and infant mental health at Wayne State University in Detroit, Michigan, and is a part-time faculty member. Mickey has maintained an Arvigo Therapy practice in Ann Arbor, Michigan, for more than 12 years because she feels that these techniques are so closely aligned with her overall interest in promoting health and recovery for all women.

A Couple's Journey to Parenthood

Give nature half a chance,
and she has a miracle in store
for everyone.

—DR. ROSITA ARVIGO

Annette   The old expression "it takes a village to raise a child"
is likely true, but my own experience tells me that the village is
involved long before the child is even born.

My husband and I had trouble getting pregnant. Between the
dreaded diagnosis of "unexplained infertility" offered by our clinic
and his male factor infertility, we were in for a ride. Prior to getting
on this ride, we made a conscious decision to prepare for it to ensure a
successful run.

Before visiting a fertility clinic (refusing to call it infertility
clinic), I was seeing a therapist for an anxiety disorder and receiving
acupuncture treatments monthly for several months, a naturopath,
and osteopath all who specialize in fertility challenges. My
experiences with these professional sessions left me feeling great!
The acupuncture decreased the anxiety, the naturopathy addressed
physical issues such as decreasing inflammatory substances in my diet,
and the osteopathy addressed structural elements that were putting a
strain on my reproductive system. I became anxiety free, energized,
and at greater peace with my struggle to conceive. After these sessions
I knew I was creating a safe happy place to carry a child beneath my
heart. I thought I was ready.

After an early miscarriage and more than one failed procedure, I wanted to add to my support network of practitioners. I wasn't sure what I was looking for and stumbled onto the Arvigo Techniques of Maya Abdominal Therapy® while browsing the Internet and wondering if I should branch out and try some of the really bizarre stuff I found since the "guaranteed" methods were not working. I found Nancy Crawford's website and became intrigued by the Arvigo Therapy, making an appointment with her that would ultimately change our lives.

The Arvigo Therapy sessions provided by Nancy provided effects I never imagined. Some were physical and others were spiritual and emotional as we worked to heal the hurts I didn't realize were there. In her capable hands I let go of negativity, embraced light and love, and felt at peace that I was gearing up to become a mother.

PRACTITIONER PERSPECTIVE   I first saw Annette in April 2012. She was 30 years old, married three years to her husband, Michael, who is 29. The couple had been trying to conceive for three years. Her initial six-month goal was to find balance and one-year goal to be pregnant. She had been taking oral contraception for 10 years and then used a Nuva ring that was removed prior to their wedding. She conceived once in September/October 2011 but subsequently miscarried that November.

They were planning an IUI procedure (intra-uterine insemination) in June 2012 which did not leave us much time to work together. She had been informed she had a "retroverted uterus with an acute anterior curve in her cervix." From her first menses at age 11 her flow had been dark red and very painful.

The tissue above her pubic bone felt full and congested more on the right side than the left, and I noted her hips and sacrum were out of alignment. I applied the Arvigo Therapy protocol as well as specialized techniques to address a retroverted uterus. Although she appeared positive and hopeful, there seemed to be an air of sadness around her. Home care instructions included the self-care massage, wearing of a faja, vaginal steam baths, herbal tonic for uterine cleansing and support, spiritual bath, and castor oil packs. Normally, I space these treatments over a few sessions, but since she was scheduled for an IUI the next month, I felt it was important to include as many as possible now.

Annette returned for her second visit 2 weeks later and reported feeling balanced and refreshed. She had just finished her period prior to this second treatment and said "this was the easiest period I have ever had!" The colour of the flow was bright red, all liquid, no clots, no pain, and she bled for five days. She smudged her home with sage and prayers, feeling a shift in energy. This session included the retroversion techniques and full Arvigo Therapy treatment. Since she was preparing for IUI later this month, we practiced visualization techniques to support a healthy conception. I recommended a pre-IUI steam of comfrey and lavender.

Annette reported the IUI procedure was awesome, feeling she was well prepared and the doctor did a great job. She left the procedure feeling positive. The morning after the procedure she experienced some cramping above the navel with light spotting.

Sadly, this IUI procedure was unsuccessful and she returned for her third treatment on July 12, 2012. She feels that although the procedure was not successful, she is in a positive frame of mind. I proceeded with the treatment session including the retroversion techniques. I noted that her pelvis was softening, muscles were releasing, and from what I could tell her uterine area felt more pliable and flexible. My recommendations included self-care massage nightly up to the fertility clinic procedure with vaginal steams the night before and morning of the IUI again with lavender and comfrey.

That same month, husband Michael scheduled a session with me. He verbalized his feelings of sadness by the "failures" in this reproductive process. While supportive of their exploration of alternative therapies, at this moment he did not share his wife's enthusiasm. He was interested in receiving energetic and spiritual healing and started seeing me routinely with his wife. He was so open to the healing process that he was able to share his feelings of sadness and hurt especially when seeing a pregnant woman or family. He saw me for two sessions and received spiritual bathing as well. His thoughts shifted to feeling more supportive and able to turn negative thinking into positive thoughts.

In August of 2012 I saw Annette one more time, continuing with the same treatment sessions as before.

She conceived and had her first ultrasound in October of that year. I continued to work with her during her pregnancy and on June 3, 2013, her baby was born in the morning.

The entire family was present for our session nine weeks postpartum. I find this is one of my favourite times, to meet the baby out of the womb. Annette received her first postpartum Arvigo Therapy session; mom and babe enjoyed a spiritual bath as well. This couple has been the most amazing to work with. Their enthusiasm, focus, and determination are commendable. I am honored and blessed to know this work from Rosita Arvigo and the traditional healers before her, including Don Elijio Panti, and to be able to assist others in this way.

Annette's Experience
I can honestly say that including Arvigo Therapy closed the circle of treatments I was receiving, balancing the purely medical therapies of the fertility clinic with other more holistic approaches. It was the missing link. It bridged body, mind, and spirit in such a way that everything became better balanced. The hands-on bodywork delivered by Nancy's magical touch penetrated my skin to help heal my soul. I left each treatment session feeling peaceful, strengthened, and whole.

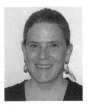

Nancy Crawford Nancy is an accomplished Reiki master/teacher, spiritual healer, and a certified Arvigo Therapy practitioner. She has also devoted more than 35 years as a registered nurse working in a variety of health care fields in Ontario and British Columbia, Canada. Her background and foundation in conventional healing led to an interest in alternative approaches, beginning with the "hands-on healing" method of Reiki, and then instinctively moving to the spiritual level of healing. Training in the wonderful ancient healing techniques began with Spiritual Healing in the rainforest of Belize, Central America, and continued on with the Arvigo Therapy studies in the United States, all under the tutelage of Rosita Arvigo, DN. Nancy welcomes women, men, and children of all ages and dis-ease into her healing practice. She practices from her home just outside of Port Colborne, Ontario, Canada.

Aligning Body, Mind, and Spirit for Conception

With faith,
everything is possible.

—DON ELIJIO PANTI

Deanna My husband, Dan, and I were both 30 years old. Married for a year, we had not yet conceived. In our naiveté, we believed that it would happen quickly and easily. However, this was not the case as the outcome was always the same: no pink plus signs or missed periods. We decided we did not want to seek the conventional medical route for fertility support; friends of mine were going that route and I heard many comments about the side effects they were experiencing. I had been working with an acupuncturist after having been diagnosed with a hormonal imbalance, PCOS (polycystic ovarian syndrome), which I felt was brought on by genetics and stress. The PCOS was under control with the help of acupuncture, but we were still not able to conceive our baby. The stress of it all was getting worse as it was interfering with my sleep; I found myself clenching my jaws at night. I thought that was due to nerves and discovered yoga provided some relief.

My menstrual cycle generally occurred on time every 33 to 34 days, with dark blood at the beginning and end of my cycle. I was charting my menstrual cycles and noted there were cycles when I did not ovulate.

Knowing how much we wanted a child, I began to investigate further all the natural modalities available for fertility enhancement and found Trish DeTura's name and website. I read about the Arvigo Techniques of Maya Abdominal Therapy® and discussed what I learned with my husband. We decided we would give it a try, so we called Trish's office, made an appointment, and drove from the Jersey Shore to her office in Hoboken one evening after work.

During our initial visit, Trish thoroughly reviewed my intake form and took the time to discuss my emotional and spiritual aspects in addition to the physical ones, noting that all aspects are addressed with Arvigo Therapy. Trish used a variety of teaching tools including diagrams of the reproductive system and uterine models; she showed me a picture of fertile cervical mucus. After listening and making some professional suggestions, Trish performed the Arvigo Therapy and taught me the self-care component. I felt good knowing I would be impacting my health by performing the self-care massage at home and hopefully conceiving sooner.

PRACTITIONER PERSPECTIVE   Deanna made the initial appointment to include both herself and her husband. Not every couple comes to the appointment together even though I request that they do so if possible. Upon entering the room, Deanna and Dan sat next to each other as we reviewed the intake form and discussed what had been shared. The love they had for one another was evident, but I noticed at the same time the stress their fertility journey was causing them.

As I began Deanna's treatment, we agreed on a centering prayer to support their faith to become parents. During the session I felt the tension in her upper abdomen and diaphragm release. My hands gently helped to encourage the uterus to move to a more central, optimal position in her pelvis. Posteriorly, her hips were misaligned, and the sacrum felt tense upon palpation.

Upon completing the session, I taught her self-care massage and jokingly told her not to worry too much about remembering the instructions because they were available on the handout we provide for our clients; we understand that sometimes a treatment relaxes you so much that it is difficult to take in much more.

While Deanna was dressing, Dan received an Arvigo Therapy session as well. His upper abdomen was also tense but slowly relaxed into my touch. He also was instructed in self-care massage because partners need just as much support and this was a great way for them to support each other.

At the close of our session I suggested Deanna and Dan share with one another why they decided to marry each other and to focus on their love for each other. Many a time, I'll ask the couple to consider doing what they did on their first date just to experience the simple joys of their lives that have been overshadowed by this fertility challenge. In addition Deanna was asked to document her basal body temperature on the charts to gain an indication for ovulation. We opted not to establish a follow-up appointment for it was already late in the evening and decided to stay in touch via phone.

While this was the only session we had together we stayed in touch via phone and e-mail. I am happy to report they are parents to a beautiful son! The combination of acupuncture, supplements, and Arvigo Therapy supported this couple's journey to become parents.

As a result of my work with this couple, I have received many referrals. Arvigo Therapy is unique in that it encompasses the mental/emotional, physical, and spiritual aspects of care that all women (and partners) deserve as they address their fertility. A major aspect of our care as Arvigo Therapy practitioners is that we address all aspects of our client's life.

Deanna's Experience

When we initially met Trish for a consultation and treatment in January of that year, she was so thorough and calming, and she explained everything to us. She gave us homework, a self-care massage, to continue at home after the treatment. We continued with the self-care massage throughout February and March. Trish made me aware of the physical, emotional, and mental attributes tied to the stomach and abdominal areas. As I continued to apply the self-care massage and took the herbal supplements, I started to feel connected to my body in a way that I hadn't before. But in March I started to get antsy and impatient and began to contemplate going for the conventional infertility treatment. Then April came and I took a pregnancy test, and it confirmed that I was indeed pregnant! After all this time of worry and concern, my prayers had been answered. Our very healthy baby boy was born the following January.

Looking back, I can honestly say that Trish and Arvigo Therapy played such an important role in my journey to conception. The treatment helped to realign us, and the self-care massage connected me to a part of my body I'd never given a second thought to before. I highly recommend Trish! You will find that is she not only an incredible practitioner, highly trained and knowledgeable, but also a compassionate and kind person. This journey can be so lonely, and regular Western medicine can be so clinical, that just talking with a caring and nurturing practitioner can give you hope, calm your spirit, and give you strength to continue to pursue the highest calling of being a mother!

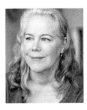

Trish DeTura RN, CNM, MS, MBT   As a certified Arvigo Therapy Practitioner and educator, Trish assists Rosita Arvigo in teaching the Advanced Pregnancy Program and has helped empower many practitioners to bring the Arvigo Techniques of Maya Abdominal Therapy® to their home communities around the world. Through her private practice, Women's Holistic Healing, in Bergen County, New Jersey, Trish enhances the lives and outcomes of couples facing fertility challenges, provides relief to women experiencing the common discomforts of pregnancy, helps women have more efficient labor and births by encouraging optimal uterine positioning, and supports women during postpartum as they heal physically, emotionally, and spiritually.

Unexplained Infertility:
Mom Knows Best

Vivian I started my TTC (trying to conceive) journey a year before I got married in February 2011. I was on birth control for 6 years prior to my wedding, and I decided to stop the birth control a year before my wedding to give my body time to detox from the medication. I made an appointment with my ob/gyn later on that year in December 2011 to get tested and make sure my body would be ready to conceive. Results came back and everything looked great.

Fast forward a year later, to May 2012, when we were excited to get started on our family. After our wedding, we decided to let nature take its course, but after three months of trying to conceive without success I began using ovulation predictor kits to detect when I was ovulating as well as fertility monitors to see if that would help. After three months of using both, we still had not conceived.

I told my mother about my inability to conceive. She shared with me her story of conceiving my brother. After I was born she wasn't able to get pregnant with her second child. At the time I was eight years old, and we took a trip to Mexico, where she told her mother (my grandmother) about her struggle to conceive her second child in spite of doing things in accordance with all the correct medical information known back then. My grandmother then told her she would give her a Mayan massage and vaginal steam bath, after which she conceived my brother right away. Mom suggested that I receive these treatments.

Not wanting to make a trip to Mexico, I searched online and found a blog from a woman who had a "Maya massage" and vaginal steam bath at the Earth & Sky Center where the Arvigo Techniques of Maya Abdominal Therapy® were offered. After receiving these treatments this woman conceived naturally.

I had my first session with Katinka Locascio in February of 2013, which was the most relaxing and optimistic experience. Imagine . . . to my amazement a month after the initial session, the pregnancy test was positive. However, I miscarried shortly after (this was referred to medically as a "chemical pregnancy"). At my second appointment in April, Katinka reassured me that my body was responding to the treatment. She gave me another Arvigo Therapy session and instructions for home self-care massage and vaginal steam baths. We planned to give it another two to three months to see if I would conceive naturally and then discuss what the next steps would be.

PRACTITIONER PERSPECTIVE Vivian came to see me because she was actively TTC for a year. She was 30 years old at the time and had been off the pill for two years. She was currently using ovulation predictor kit sticks to better time her fertile window. She shared the story of her mother's challenge to conceive her brother. When she learned that I was an Arvigo Therapy practitioner and that vaginal steams *(bajos)* are part of the session, she came to see me.

At the first visit we reviewed her intake form and noted she had dark blood at the beginning of her cycle, painful periods, water retention, bloating, and low back discomfort—all symptoms of stagnation. Vivian had been charting her cycle and had a clear ovulatory pattern with at least 12 high temperatures in her luteal phase.

On the first visit we did a complete anterior treatment as well as a steam. The massage revealed a clear pattern of emotional holding in the lower abdomen. Her womb was generally centered though somewhat anterior leaning. We discussed doing daily self-care massage or warm hands and monthly steams. I also suggested some dietary guidelines to help reduce the water retention and prepare her body for a pregnancy.

Our second visit was rescheduled because Vivian called me to let me know she had had a chemical pregnancy that month. She had done her self-care (warm hands) and her period was late. A pregnancy test gave a faint line, which lessened each day, until finally her menses started; this time her menses started with bright red blood.

At Vivian's second Arvigo Therapy session in April, we added to her at home self-care regimen as her uterus felt much more open, and the emotional holding had shifted. I recommended doing the steams at home for the next few months, continuing with self-care massage and a tea with nettle, raspberry leaf, oats, and red clover.

Vivian's Experience

In May I still hadn't conceived and decided to schedule an appointment with fertility specialists for July "just in case." I did not need that appointment as the next month, June, I was pregnant. I was overjoyed with the news! I truly believe that Arvigo Therapy, self care, and vaginal steam baths helped me to finally conceive.

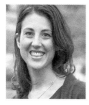

Katinka Locascio LMT (www.earthandskyhealingarts.com) Katinka is a licensed massage therapist in New York state, herbalist, body worker, and labor doula. She founded Earth & Sky Healing Arts 10 years ago with a vision to helping people live to their fullest potential while staying rooted in the wisdom of the body. Inspired by her background in science, she has pursued numerous trainings in the healing arts. Her practice focuses on women's health, pregnancy, and fertility, as well as integrative structural bodywork. She is currently pursuing a degree in osteopathic manual therapy and is looking forward to starting her two-year research dissertation. She lives and works in Long Island City, Queens, New York.

Infertility   The inability to acheive pregnancy after 12 months of trying to conceive is defined as infertility. Approximately 10 percent of the population is affected; 30 percent of infertility can be attributed to male factors and about 30 percent can be attributed to female factors. In about 20 percent of cases infertility is unexplained, and the remaining 10 percent is caused by a combination of problems in both partners. Common causes of female infertility include ovulation problems (PCOS), fallopian tube blockage, pelvic inflammatory disease, uterine problems, endometriosis, and age-related factors. The main cause of male infertility is low semen quality (count, morphology, motility) and in some cases testicular malformation, hormone imbalance, or blocked ducts. In cases of unexplained infertility, it is believed that abnormalities are likely present but not detectable by current methods. Infertility testing involves a complete medical history and physical examination of both partners; blood work (hormones, thyroid function); and imaging tests (pelvic ultrasound, hysterosalpingogram, or HSG, and laparoscopy) for women and sperm analysis for men. Treatment depends on the cause of infertility. It may involve education and counseling, medication, surgery, fertility treatments such as intrauterine insemination (IUI), and in vitro fertilization (IVF). As many as one in five couples diagnosed with infertility eventually become pregnant without treatment. More than half of couples with infertility become pregnant after treatment.

Renewed Hope for Conception as Fallopian Tube Blockage Resolves

When it's dark enough,
you can see the stars.

—RALPH WALDO EMERSON

Karla I'm in my late thirties and I have been experiencing menstrual cycles with low back pain along with a pulling sensation in the back area for some time now. Cycles are regular so I can plan on when the pain is going to begin. For a couple of years we have been trying to conceive without success. Due to increased back pain I consulted with my ob/gyn, who recommended an abdominal laparoscopic procedure to determine the cause of the pain. The procedure was extended to 4 hours of surgery when severe endometriosis and endometrial adhesions were found. My left fallopian tube was completely blocked with endometriosis, which was most likely a source of my fertility challenges. I was told that this would always remain blocked; there was nothing that could be done. My right fallopian tube was open. My doctor said my uterus was retroverted, but she stated that the uterus position was likely not causing my pain or inability to conceive. Regardless, they were not aware of a way to alter the position of the uterus.

After the surgery I had less back pain with my periods. Although I wasn't instructed by my medical care providers on any follow-up actions I could do to improve my blocked fallopian tube, I decided to improve my diet after reading articles about how important nutrient-dense, anti-inflammatory foods are for maintaining good health. I also started working with an acupuncturist and began an exercise program. In my search for additional things I could add to my wellness program, I was intrigued when I read about the Arvigo Techniques of Maya Abdominal Therapy® on the Internet and was delighted to find Heidi Jost, a certified Arvigo practitioner, whose office was not far from where I lived.

PRACTITIONER PERSPECTIVE   When Karla came to see me, she reported that she was experiencing fertility challenges and had extensive endometrial surgery and a blocked fallopian tube. Even though her surgery was recent, her periods were becoming painful again; she was having significant blood clotting and cramping while menstruating. She was also experiencing occasional stress incontinence. When I assessed her lower abdomen, I found that her uterus was low and left, which was also the side of the fallopian tube blockage. Karla had an initial 2-hour session and was taught the self-care massage to perform as per instructions at home. Because of her painful cramping and fertility challenges I also included castor oil packs in her plan.

I worked with Karla twice a month for almost a year. During this time, Karla continued to work with her acupuncturist on a regular basis, maintained an impeccable diet, and utilized castor oil packs. It was apparent in our sessions that Karla's dedication and diligence in doing her self care was having positive results.

Karla's Experience   I could not believe how wonderful my
body felt after I would do my self-care massage. I was also amazed at how healthy my periods were, no longer painful or clotty, and my stress incontinence had ceased. However, after a year of multifaceted dedication, I still was not pregnant. I returned to my ob/gyn for some follow-up tests. I had a hysterosalpingogram (HSG) to check if my tubes were patent [unobstructed] or if there was more endometriosis. The doctor said the results revealed no reason I couldn't conceive, as both my fallopian tubes were patent, my uterus was in normal

position, and there was no sign of endometriosis. She did not remember the blockage so when I mentioned it and she compared HSG results, she was speechless. She was unable to explain how my left fallopian tube became unblocked or how my endometriosis was no longer present. She emphasized that the uterus was in normal position and both fallopian tubes were patent, and that was positive for me.

I knew these changes in my body had happened because of the positive steps I was taking and this brought me renewed hope about future conception success. I am so thankful for having experienced Arvigo Therapy and learning the self-care massage techniques and assistive modalities. Hopeful, I continue to do the self-care massage along with pursuing other natural fertility enhancement methods.

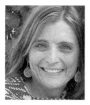 **Heidi Marie Jost** RN, NKH, LP, CH (www.theessentialconnection.net) Heidi, an integrated holistic practitioner, has been a registered nurse for 31 years, a clinical perfusionist for 22 years, a nondual healer for 12 years, and a chartered herbalist for 16 years. She has 16 years of experience with the Arvigo Techniques of Maya Abdominal Therapy® and is a certified practitioner, certified Self Care teacher, and a certified Pregnancy practitioner. Heidi pursues her passion for advanced healing through the exploration of the essential connection of mind, heart, and body. She believes in helping her clients develop a deeper awareness through self care to harness the potential that exists within to promote healing and improve quality of life. Heidi has offices in Illinois and Wisconsin.

Overcoming Secondary Infertility after Caesarean Birth

When the world says,
"Give up," Hope whispers,
"Try one more time."

—ANONYMOUS

Sydney   It was easy conceiving our first child. In 2008, we decided we were ready to start a family. We had been together since high school, married for two years, and I was 24 years old. It took four months, and voila! We were pregnant and now have a beautiful son born on Halloween 2009. So how could I be affected by infertility now? My son was born by caesarean section after hours of laboring and pushing. I never knew what a profound impact a c-section would have on our ability to have more children, and what an emotional roller coaster it would be for me trying to conceive our second child.

A big family has been a dream of ours so we started trying to conceive when my son was just a few months old. Why not keep up the momentum? This time it took a bit longer to get pregnant, but since I was breast feeding a year didn't seem unreasonable. A few weeks later, we had a miscarriage and were completely devastated; it shook up our entire world.

We spent a lot of time healing after that, and asked a lot of "why" questions. Many women I talked to who also had miscarried at some point assured me that we would likely be pregnant again in no time. While I was fine with a little bit of time passing first to continue the emotional and physical healing process of losing that baby, I was definitely still anxious to keep growing our family. And then there was month after month of negative pregnancy tests. Half a year later, I decided that it was finally time to seek help and soon after learned about secondary infertility. At times I felt I would never conceive again, and it was hard just to not give up.

I met another yoga mama here in Austin who is a wealth of knowledge of all things fertility-related. Not only did I get to partake in her wonderful three-month Yoga for Fertility course with a group of other beautiful women on their own fertility journeys, but she also connected me with two other women who now play an important role in my life. One is the acupuncturist I see for weekly treatments to enhance my fertility, and she makes sure I'm taking the right combination of Chinese herbs to further assist. The second woman is Charlotte Westbrook, a clinical massage therapist who is a certified practitioner of the Arvigo Techniques of Maya Abdominal Therapy®. What Charlotte taught me and continues to do for me every month is invaluable. I feel completely blessed to have discovered this support network of amazing women who are helping me heal.

Charlotte discovered there was a lot of scar tissue and adhesions in my abdomen from the c-section. My uterus was not in an ideal position where it could receive proper blood flow and nutrients, and this was having a significant impact on my healing and optimal postpartum reproductive functioning. Charlotte treated me with Arvigo Therapy to help my uterus reposition itself. She also taught me some great self-care massage to do at home between our sessions in addition to using castor oil packs at the beginning of my cycle. The Arvigo Therapy also greatly assisted me with releasing the emotional trauma related to both my c-section birth and subsequent miscarriage.

PRACTITIONER PERSPECTIVE   When Syndey entered my office, I couldn't help but smile. She was one of those sweet, heartfelt, bubbly personalities mixed with sheer determination. The excitement she felt about receiving this work was contagious. Under the surface, however, there was palpable sadness and deep grief. She told me of her longings to have a large family and the birth story of her first child. Her ideal birth plan hadn't turned out as planned: She ended up having a c-section after being in labor for 18 hours and pushing for two hours. Her frustration and anger at this outcome was understandable. Eighteen months after her first child was born, Syndey was able to get pregnant again and shortly thereafter had a miscarriage. As Syndey's story continued to unfold, I could feel the deep-seated grief that only the loss of a child can evoke in a person. Her physical symptoms included dark, thick blood at the beginning of her cycle, headaches and bloating with her period, emotional mood swings, and low backache at the beginning of her cycle.

Expecting to find scar tissue from the c-section, I started the first session with a castor oil pack and started every subsequent session with a castor oil pack either to the abdomen or the sacrum. While the castor oil was working its magic, I did some craniosacral work to ease Sydney into the session and get her used to my energy and touch. Her uterine position was difficult to detect in the first few sessions due to the scar tissue, but I sensed the fundus low and to the right. Sydney's pelvic bones were unbalanced and her sacrum was holding more tension on one side than the other. I taught Sydney self-care massage and sent her home with some guidelines for natural fertility enhancement during each part of her cycle. I also instructed her on how, when, and where to apply castor oil packs at home.

Our first two sessions were primarily focused on releasing the external scar tissue, and releasing the muscular tension that was contributing to her pelvis's misalignment. The headaches and bloating were relieved after these initial sessions. The third session was a tandem session where another skilled practitioner was invited to join in the healing process at Sydney's request to receive energy healing as a complement to Arvigo Therapy. Sydney claims that this most recent session helped her to release the remaining grief associated with her miscarriage and to begin the release of emotions that were associated with the birth of her son.

In my experience working with women post c-section, scars can be particulary complicated because there is external scar tissue from the orignal incision, and scarring where the uterus was cut open to safely remove the new-born. The obstetrical surgeon's main concern during this process is making the delivery as fast and efficient as possible for safety and health reasons, but the position in which the uterus is returned to the body after the baby's removal can have an impact on the way the body heals. The body also has a way of storing emotions from traumatic events into associated areas of the body.

As Sydney's body healed from the surgery, it took me a few sessions to figure out the status of her uterus as it seemed the fundus was shifted low and to the right of the pelvis, which is something I see quite often, but in between each session it had found its way back over there and quickly started to lay down adhesions again. I included side-lying techniques with the hope this would release some of the adhesions. This session and the next one were focused on releasing the adhesions that were causing the constriction in the lower pelvis. This enabled her uterus to easily glide into a more ideal position, and her low back and hip pain cleared as a result. During our seventh session we focused more on helping to stabilize her lower back and pelvis. After this session Sydney reported that the dark clotting during her menses had finally resolved. Our final session together was another tandem session with another practitioner, which was primarily a maintenance session full of joy.

Sydney and I worked together for a total of eight sessions for the better part of a year. The entire process from the first session to the last was a constant interplay of physical, emotional, and energetic releases. Each energetic and emotional release allowed her body to release more of the physical scar tissue and tension. As her uterus eased its way into a more ideal position, her emotions also started to stabilize. Her dedication to her own healing process was essential as each time we reached a new layer of scarring, there would be an emotional component that had to be acknowledged and then released.

Sydney's Experience

I spent the better part of a year focusing on my health, improving my fertility, and doing everything I could to make sure my body was in tiptop shape for another pregnancy. I continued with Arvigo Therapy sessions with Charlotte about once a month, self-care massage and castor oil packs regularly at home, weekly acupuncture treatments and Chinese herbs to help with hormone balancing, a regular yoga practice, and healthy eating.

Our family decided to do something out of the ordinary since pregnancy wasn't happening. We decided to pack up and travel. While traveling I tried to remove myself from everything I was doing during that year's quest for pregnancy and just not think about it. While our months of traveling had their ups and downs and were far from a "vacation," overall it was a great experience that I would never trade for anything. We gained a lot of perspective as to who we were as individuals and as a family. We wouldn't have become who we are now without those experiences. We became such a tight-knit family unit that nothing—not even unemployment, a dwindling bank account, and no place to live—could destroy.

Four months later, as I was searching through my suitcase, I came across an unopened pregnancy test that I had been toting around since we left Austin. What a surprise when those two pink lines showed up. It was positive, and I was finally pregnant!

I honestly feel like I couldn't have arrived at that positive pregnancy test without all of the steps I took to prepare my body and mind to get there. I also feel like it happened when it was supposed to and only after I truly let go of some of the emotions I was holding. We were ecstatic, and as I sit here at 22 weeks pregnant expecting another baby boy, I'm savoring every single second of this pregnancy that I never thought I'd be graced with. My journey to get to this point, being pregnant with another healthy baby, has taught me much. And I am *so* grateful for all of it. I have learned more about my body, my health, my fertility, and myself than I had ever imagined I would.

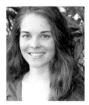

Charlotte Westbrook BS, LMTI (www.charlotteshealinghands.com) Charlotte is a licensed massage therapist in both Texas and Maine and a certified Self Care instructor and practitioner for the Arvigo Techniques of Maya Abdominal Therapy®. She also specializes in craniosacral therapy and customized pain-relief sessions. The core belief in her practice is that the body naturally wants to heal itself, and her job is to help create the space for that healing to occur. Charlotte works to bring the body into alignment through time-honored massage techniques that are tailored for individual needs, while incorporating craniosacral therapy, Maya Spiritual Healing, and Reiki to be able to address emotional and spiritual blocks. She is also starting a nonprofit organization, Safe Contact, that will offer empowerment workshops and lecture series to people who have been sexually, physically, emotionally, or spiritually abused.

Secondary Infertility   The inability to become pregnant, or to carry a pregnancy to term, following the birth of one or more biological children, is known as secondary infertility. The rising rate of secondary infertility, which has increased 60 percent since 1995, is thought to be caused by the increasing number of couples waiting until they are older and more financially stable to have children, as well as couples in second or third marriages who decide to have another child. Many couples who conceived a first child easily are stunned to find themselves unable to conceive a second child. According to Resolve, the National Fertility Association, secondary infertility is more common than primary infertility. Common causes of secondary infertility are age, weight gain, ovulation problems, endometriosis, pelvic adhesions, uterine fibroids or polyps, infection from previous childbirth, D&C, or c-section. Asherman's syndrome (intrauterine adhesions as a result of scarring after uterine surgery) is seen in women who have been pregnant, and research has shown that c-sections can cause infertility for 1 in 3 women. In addition, partner's sperm count, motility, or health may have deteriorated, or there may be impotence or ejaculation problems. Suffering secondary infertility can be particularly difficult emotionally for couples; they may feel guilty for not providing a sibling for their other child, selfish for delaying a second pregnancy until it was "too late" to conceive, or for not being content with just one child.

Self Care Enhances Assisted Reproductive Technology Outcome

Our bodies are our gardens to
which our wills are gardeners.

—WILLIAM SHAKESPEARE

Julia After over four years of trying to conceive through ART
(assisted reproductive technology) without success, I began to seek
alternative supportive therapies to assist my husband and me on our
quest to have a baby. I had heard of "Maya massage," eventually
leading me to the Arvigo Techniques of Maya Abdominal Therapy®
and Beth Townsend. After reading about the modality and the
benefits, we decided to set up a session with Beth.

PRACTITIONER PERSPECTIVE Julia scheduled a session as she prepared for
her fourth round of IVF (in vitro fertilization). She had been unable to hold
the previous transfers as her uterine lining never increased beyond eight mm of
thickness with conventional medicine. This was going to be her final attempt
at conception after several years of assisted reproductive technology including
IUI (intra uterine insemination) and IVF cycles.

In her initial session it felt like her uterus was positioned low in the pelvic bowl, leaning forward (anterior) and with more fullness to the right. Her
hips were misaligned, with sacral tension and congestion present. During this
session I could feel her uterus gently shifting and less congestion in this area

84

afterward. Her back and sacral alignment improved, and she felt relief from the pressure she had been accustomed to.

In addition to the bodywork session, we discussed the impact of stress, long-distance driving for her work, dietary changes, and other supportive stress-management techniques. She was instructed in home self-care massage that would improve circulation to the digestive and reproductive organs. Our treatment plan was to schedule practitioner sessions every other week, daily self care, dietary changes, and swimming, which she enjoyed.

On her second visit Julia reported an improvement in elimination and digestion as well as a decrease in her low back pain and attributed this to the swimming several times per week. Her uterus still felt low and to the right, but with less congestion than at the initial session. Given her sacral area was still congested and tense, a castor oil pack was applied to help address this during the session as well as becoming part of her home care routine.

Her third session was scheduled just after her menstrual cycle, which was different than what she was used to. There was less cramping than during previous cycles; flow was bright red blood instead of dark brown; and the cycle was five days instead of the usual seven. These were significant changes, and Julia was delighted. I noted that her uterus was still low, but more centered in the pelvic bowl and less congested. Her hips were in better alignment and the sacrum was less congested and tense.

Julia was due to return to her fertility specialist for the process of preparing for her final IVF treatment. Our treatment plan included ongoing self-care massage and castor oil packs rotating between abdomen and sacrum. We discussed the benefits of vaginal steams, but with her busy schedule it would be "next to impossible."

We were able to have two more sessions in the process of preparation for IVF, with the final visit occurring five days prior to egg retrieval. She called me to report her uterine lining had increased to 11 mm at the time of transfer. Two weeks later pregnancy was confirmed with twins. When she was 20 weeks I began applying the Arvigo Therapy prenatal protocol and continued it throughout the rest of her pregnancy until the twins were born at 35½ weeks (twin B was growing slowly).

Julia's Experience

What an amazing journey to motherhood with Arvigo Therapy and Beth. Throughout our sessions I would leave feeling lighter and more balanced. Doing the self-care massage at home gave me something to do that was relaxing and nurturing as I imagined my uterine lining becoming thick and ready for our baby. It was amazing to see my uterine lining increase to 11 mm as we prepared for the transfer; this had never happened before! I saw Beth throughout my pregnancy and had a minimal amount of digestive issues and low back pain. We are now the proud parents of twins—a boy and a girl—and loving every minute of it.

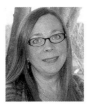

Beth Ann Townsend MMT, HHP (http://bethanntownsend.com/) Beth Ann has a thriving practice in Grand Rapids, Michigan, where she serves her clients with the Arvigo Techniques of Maya Abdominal Therapy® including advanced training in Pregnancy, from preconception through post partum. She assists families, men, women, and children with treatment and education so they feel empowered to make better choices for themselves. Beth Ann has studied complementary health practices from indigenous cultures since the early '70s and has integrated into her practice craniosacral therapy, manual therapy, medical massage, herbal and organic whole food nutrition education, and energy therapies, including healing touch, Reiki, and Touch for Health. Beth Ann is a certified Arvigo instructor offering the Hands on Health the Maya Way and Self Care training.

Assisted Reproductive Technology (ART)   The processes of surgically removing eggs from a woman's ovaries, combining them with sperm in the laboratory, and returning them to the woman's body or donating them to another woman, are known as assisted reproductive technology (ART). Common methods of ART include in vitro fertilization (IVF), the most widely used and considered the most effective; zygote intrafallopian transfer (ZIFT) or tubal embryo transfer; gamete intrafallopian transfer (GIFT), where eggs and sperm are transferred into the woman's fallopian tube and fertilization occurs in the woman's body; and intracytoplasmic sperm injection (ICSI), in which a single sperm is injected into a mature egg versus the sperm fertilizing the egg on its own (often used for couples with male factor infertility). ART procedures sometimes involve the use of donor eggs, donor sperm, or previously frozen embryos. An infertile woman or couple may also use donor embryos; the child will not be genetically related to either parent. Success rates vary and depend on many factors, including the clinic performing the procedure, the infertility diagnosis, and the age of the woman undergoing the procedure. According to the Centers for Disease Control (CDC) the average percentage of fresh, non-donor ART cycles that led to a live birth ranged from 40 percent in women younger than 35 years of age down to 22 percent in women aged 38 to 40 and only 1 percent in women 44 years and older. ART can be expensive and time-consuming, but it has allowed many couples to have children that otherwise would not have been conceived. It is worth noting that a recent major study into the health of newborns found that children born after IVF treatment have a greater risk of complications ranging from preterm birth to neonatal death; doctors found that single IVF babies were nearly twice as likely to be born early, to be stillborn, or to die within the first 28 days of delivery compared with those conceived naturally.

Conception Success in Spite of Polycystic Ovarian Syndrome

*We delight in the beauty of
the butterfly, but rarely admit
the changes it has gone through
to achieve that beauty.*

—MAYA ANGELOU

Abigail   At 24 years old I had a history of headaches, skin problems, and cramping with menses for some time. The doctor had told me that since I had polycystic ovarian syndrome (PCOS) I would probably never get pregnant and if I did I would most likely miscarry. I tried birth control pills and an IUD to prevent getting pregnant so that I wouldn't experience a potential miscarriage. I began having constant bleeding and cramping when the IUD had been in for six months. Although the doctor insisted that it was unrelated, I had the IUD removed. The bleeding stopped in six days, but the cramping continued. I then looked for more natural ways to help with my bleeding and cramping and found a local Arvigo Techniques of Maya Abdominal Therapy® practitioner.

At my initial session, Lorraine Paquette showed me how to perform the self-care massage techniques to support the health of my uterus and ovaries. I began doing this abdominal massage about four times a week and within a month was feeling clearer and calmer. Lorraine added an herbal tincture to my home program and by the next month I had a normal period without cramping or clumps in my flow. I also had no further headaches. I continued to have treatments with Lorraine about once a month and my cycles continued to improve, until at 6 months into this program I became pregnant. When I went to see Lorraine she adjusted my self care for my pregnancy and I continued to see her on occasion during the pregnancy for my health and to address my hip pain. I had a healthy baby boy!

PRACTITIONER PERSPECTIVE   When Abigail came for her first Arvigo Therapy visit, her concerns were cramping with her periods and persistent bleeding. She had had her IUD removed and recently stopped flowing after almost 2 months of continuous bleeding but was still having painful cramping. She would exercise regularly and watch her diet to keep her weight under control.

Her treatment included the Arvigo Techniques of Maya Abdominal Therapy® with massage to her back and abdominal areas. Her low back muscles were tight and she was tender over the sacrum and adjacent areas. Tenderness was present in multiple abdominal areas. Her uterus was felt to be positioned high and to the right. She was taught to do the self-care techniques and reported feeling "good" after her first treatment.

Abigail continued to have treatments about once a month and reported decreased bloating, without pain or clotting, with the next few periods. Her headaches went away and cravings for sweets were decreased during this time as well. Within 6 months she successfully conceived and continued treatments less often to support her uterine heath and decrease hip pain during pregnancy. Eight weeks after having her baby she returned for therapy for back pain. After this treatment she reported that she again felt great.

Abigail's Experience   Over time and since I was doing better, I forgot about doing the self care and using the Female Tonic.

A couple of years later I noticed symptoms of skin problems, was feeling depressed and emotional, and had difficulty handling stress especially around the time my period had returned. I went back to see Lorraine. Within a month I began noticing a decrease in these symptoms. I have found that monthly Arvigo Therapy sessions with Lorraine, the self-care massage, and the herbal support work together to keep my symptoms under control. My skin still breaks out sometimes but less often, and I am now able to notice the relationship of my skin condition to diet or stress in my life. As of this writing I am happy to report I am carrying my second child.

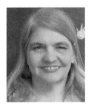 **Lorraine Paquette** MAEd, OTR/L, CHT, LMT, CLT   Lorraine is an occupational therapist and massage therapist in private practice at Mariposa Therapies in Phoenix, Arizona. In addition to the Arvigo Techniques of Maya Abdominal Therapy®, Lorraine specializes in hand therapy, lymph drainage, and visceral manipulation. She combines a variety of techniques to help people with decreasing pain, increasing the ability to perform normal activities, or to improve health, especially of the digestive, reproductive, and elimination systems. As a certified Arvigo Therapy Self Care instructor, Lorraine enjoys sharing the benefits of this work with her clients and with small groups.

Polycystic Ovary Syndrome (PCOS)   Unbalanced female hormones can cause poly-cystic ovary syndrome (PCOS). Most women with PCOS grow many small cysts on their ovaries, thus its name. The cysts are not harmful, but the hormone imbalances can cause menstrual cycle changes, difficulty conceiving, and other health changes. PCOS may also cause unwanted changes in the way a woman looks (acne, extra facial and body hair, weight gain, thinning hair on scalp). Women with PCOS often have a problem with insulin resistance. When the body doesn't use insulin well, blood sugar levels go up and over time, this increases a woman's chance of developing diabetes. PCOS is common, affecting as many as 10 percent of women aged 12 to 45 years old. Often the symptoms begin in the teen years. PCOS seems to run in families, so a woman's chance of having it is higher if other women in her family have had PCOS. There is a variety of treatments to address PCOS, each tailored to specific symptoms, presence of health problems, and whether or not the woman is trying to get pregnant. Combi-nation birth control pills are used for long-term treatment for PCOS women who do not wish to become pregnant. For those who are trying to conceive, insulin sensitizing drugs used for diabetes are prescribed. Along with weight loss and ovulation medications the treatment can help to enhance fertility. Surgery on the ovaries has been used when these other methods aren't working, but the long-term effects of this procedure are unknown. Treatment can help control PCOS symptoms and prevent long-term problems; if not treated, over time serious health problems such as diabetes and heart disease may develop.

Prenatal Wellness, Birth, and Postpartum Recovery

Pregnancy Doesn't Have to Be Painful

Your work is to discover your world and then with all your heart give yourself to it.

—BUDDHA

Heather I was about 16 weeks into my first pregnancy when I began to have lower right quadrant abdominal pain that was intermittent and spasmodic in nature. Since both my husband and I were naturopathic physicians, we started treating the pain with homeopathic remedies, but the pain worsened. One episode was so painful that I fell to my knees gasping for air. I immediately contacted my midwife (also a naturopathic physician). After she examined me and wasn't able to rule out major pathologies, I was sent to the ER for further evaluation. Our biggest concerns included appendicitis and possible ovarian torsion.

At the ER I was evaluated by sonogram and I had blood work as well. No doctor ever palpated me manually. I left the ER without a diagnosis, but with the scary possible pathologies ruled out. It was so painful to walk. I was scared of such intense pain, feeling that it would overwhelm my sense of well-being during my pregnancy and make it impossible for me to work. Right after the hospital appointment, my midwife got me an appointment with Sarah Wylie, ND, and a practitioner of the Arvigo Techniques of Maya Abdominal Therapy®.

PRACTITIONER PERSPECTIVE   I received the midwife's call updating me on Heather's condition and experience in the emergency room and was relieved to know that all of the worst case scenario conditions had been ruled out. I saw Heather in my clinic and observed her as she walked toward me in short steps, with an ashen face and walking somewhat sideways. "Antalgic posture," I thought to myself as I eased her down the hall to my treatment room. Assisting her to the exam table, I placed her in a side-lying position of comfort while I learned more about her condition. The pain had been intermittent for about 10 days and constant during the past 24 hours.

I began the Arvigo Therapy session by gently performing the lower abdominal strokes, feeling her relax under my hands. It was evident her uterus was tilted toward the right with the pelvic bones out of alignment. She had dense fibrous tissue around her posterior hips (ASIS). Upon questioning, Heather recalled she was born with congenital hip dysplasia and had been treated surgically for this. She wasn't quite sure about the extent of the surgical treatment because her mother hadn't really understood the problem or treatment well enough to explain it to her. At this initial session I also taught Heather how to self-care massage her growing belly to help keep her uterus supported in an upright and balanced position. By the time the treatment was over, Heather reported that she felt 80 percent better. By the next day, she let me know she felt 100 percent better.

Within the week, Heather had another episode. But without the fear, her pain didn't escalate as high. I got her into the clinic as soon as I could, and the same positive response to the Arvigo Therapy treatment occurred. We decided to book her in for weekly treatments. She was doing her self-care massage diligently but seemed to also benefit from the full Arvigo Therapy treatment. Heather continued to have these episodes of pain, but the interval between them spaced out such that by the time she was 24 weeks, she no longer experienced the pain. We found that the use of a faja or a pregnancy support belt called the "prenatal cradle mini" was also instrumental in keeping her from episodes of pain.

I was in attendance when Heather gave birth at home naturally at 42 weeks, induced by acupuncture and giving birth 3 hours later. She told me that having me there, after all the weeks I had given her relief from pain, helped her to relax and trust her powerful birthing sensations and yield.

Heather's Experience

Without Arvigo Therapy my pregnancy would have been clouded by fear and pain. I truly believe that working with Sarah helped prepare me physically, spiritually, and emotionally to have a triumphant, empowering birth at 41 years old. Whenever I hear pregnant women describing their pains, I tell them that they may not have to endure the pain. I refer them to an Arvigo practitioner. But I wonder how often my advice is disregarded since the prevalent belief is that pregnancy is uncomfortable. My pregnancy was such an empowering experience for me, and I believe I was able to share those feelings of "rightness" in my body with my son while he was gestating. I am forever grateful to have had an Arvigo practitioner confident working with pregnant women to nurture me back to myself. My birth was amazing, and I shall cherish those memories for my lifetime. My son was able to be born without intervention, in a room full of joy.

PRACTITIONER NOTE   In the early weeks of treatment Heather and I wove a story together about her pain. We hypothesized her body had formed scar tissue from the hip surgery as a way to stabilize her hip with some of the scar tissue adhering to the broad and round ligaments. It was most painful between 16 and 24 weeks. As her uterus grew with the baby, the scar tissue had to stretch beyond its capacity and was tearing. The fibrotic tissue was interfering with her ligamentous relaxin-induced laxity. Since this experience I have had the occasion to work with other women who have scar tissue on the ligaments, and this same time frame (16 to 24 weeks) seems to apply.

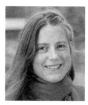

Sarah e Wylie ND (www.RedBlossomMedicine.com)   Sarah is a naturopathic doctor and midwife in the Champlain Valley of Vermont. Specializing in fertility treatment, she is passionate about helping women conceive, whether implementing a holistic approach or as a complement to conventional reproductive medicine. Sarah uses her skills in midwifery to treat women with healthy as well as complicated pregnancies through her training in the Arvigo Techniques of Maya Abdominal Therapy®. One of her goals is to empower people to feel at home in their bodies. Therefore, Arvigo Therapy is an essential piece of postpartum restoration. Sarah has enjoyed apprenticeship to Rosita Arvigo since 1998, and has taught with the Arvigo Institute since 2009.

Persistence Pays Off:
Finding Relief for Pregnancy Pain

Let your heart guide you. It
whispers, so listen carefully.

—LITTLE FOOT'S MOTHER
IN *LAND BEFORE TIME*

Kyra Beginning some time after my 20th week of pregnancy, I started
to feel like my pelvic bones were tumbling out of place every time I
sat or lay down. After a few weeks, the pain was so intense that I was
having trouble standing up in the morning to get out of bed. I began
to feel like a cartoon character, whose skeleton could be shaken up
inside but whose body could continue to lurch forward, halting and
stopping, until the bones shifted back into place. I eventually gained
more mobility during the day as I moved around, but the pain was
still there.

In hopes of finding relief, I searched the Internet, spoke with
other moms, and talked to another midwife in the practice where I
received my care. The response I received was universal: This kind
of thing happens during pregnancy, there's nothing that can be done,
and it should resolve after the birth. I was only a little over halfway
through my pregnancy, but there seemed to be no other option. I
willed myself to focus on thoughts of autumn, when the baby would
arrive and I would not wake up in increasingly severe pain.

At my next appointment with the midwives I met Anne Hirsch,
and I explained to her what was happening. To my great surprise, she

told me there might be something she could do to help. She was also a practitioner of the Arvigo Techniques of Maya Abdominal Therapy®. I lay down on the exam table and as she worked with me, it felt like she pulled my bones back into place. I felt instant relief; for the first time in weeks, I was able to walk around and stand on one foot without any pain. It was an incredibly freeing feeling. Physically, I felt as though a huge weight had been lifted off my body, and I could suddenly move again.

PRACTITIONER PERSPECTIVE   Kyra was an attorney—and a strong, competent, accomplished woman—who was pregnant for the first time. She arrived at her prenatal visit looking a little pale and moving slowly. She had to sit down oh-so-carefully. When she began to talk about the pain in her hips and groin, her eyes misted up ever so slightly. This pelvic pain was taking a toll on her. I suggested an Arvigo Therapy session might be helpful and she agreed to try it.

During the session I focused primarily on helping her relax her abdomen and rebalancing her hips and she began to experience relief right away. The most telling indicator came when she got off the table: She practically began dancing around the room as she could move freely with less pain.

This was not the first time I had seen a pregnant woman experience such great relief after Arvigo Therapy. Before I was trained in these techniques I would tell my patients, "Once your baby is born, all this will resolve." Now I have something to offer in. the moment to provide relief. Arvigo Therapy is truly a boon for a midwife who cares to help her clients when they have discomfort in pregnancy. It is also a boon for women who want to enjoy pregnancy rather than suffer through with aches and pains.

Kyra's Experience   I worked with Anne a couple more times during my pregnancy to help keep any resurgence of the pain at bay. While I felt a little stiff in the mornings throughout my pregnancy, and still had minor pain on occasions, the debilitating pain never returned. Prior to receiving Arvigo Therapy, I had never experienced massage or bodywork, or been to a chiropractor, and frankly, would

not have expected something like this to work. However, it made a huge difference in my pregnancy, and I am grateful I was lucky enough to have a midwife who was skilled in these techniques.

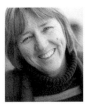 **Anne L. Hirsch** CPM, LM(WA/FL) Anne is a certified professional midwife licensed in the states of Washington and Florida and a certified Self Care teacher with the Arvigo Institute. She uses the Arvigo Techniques of Maya Abdominal Therapy® in her midwifery practice to help ease pregnancy discomforts, correct misaligned uteri, and aid recovery after the birth. She also works with women preparing before they become pregnant and those needing to heal other female concerns. Her main focus is to teach women the Self Care techniques, putting into their own hands the power to help their bodies heal. Anne currently practices in the Seattle area.

Self Care Fosters Self Love:
Healing from a Traumatic Birth

*When we give ourselves
compassion, we are opening
our hearts in a way that can
transform our lives.*

—KRISTIN NEFF

Emma We married in June 2008 and wanted to start a family right away. Three months later we were expecting our first baby! I was fairly healthy and physically active and had just quit my high-stress job to be a home health nurse so I could focus on starting a family. Since I was a nurse and worked in an ob/gyn office for 3 years, I assumed I would just show up at the hospital, get an epidural, and have a baby. However, working in pediatric home health I was exposed to babies that had suffered trauma during birth. I started doing my homework and I felt that a natural birth would be best for me and my baby. When I told my ob/gyn, he thought I was silly. I blew him off, thinking to myself, "Well, I will just show him." I pored over information on natural births (of course skipping over any c-section info since I was not having a c-section) and felt that my experience was going to be a piece of cake. I was looking forward to sharing my natural birth story with everyone.

A few days past my due date I started to pass large clots in the evening. I called my ob/gyn and was directed to go to the hospital for an examination, where I was informed my water had broken and that I was in labor. Although I was not having contractions, I was admitted. Throughout the night, hospital staff kept coming in the room, checking my dilation, looking at the fetal monitor. The doctors and nurses kept warning me that my body was not going into active labor on its own: If I did not progress soon, a Pitocin drip would be started. During an exam one of the doctors broke my water (without informing me), which made me question, "Wait a moment . . . hadn't I been told that my water had already broken?" Since the birth was not progressing, Pitocin was started and from there everything spun out of control with procedures being performed without discussion. Exhausted and nervous, I just did what the doctors told me to do rather than ask questions. I felt they knew better than me since my body did not know how to have a baby correctly.

Pitocin caused me to dilate from 3 to 10 cm in less than 45 minutes; but the baby did not drop. I suspected he was anterior facing due to the extreme back labor I was having but was informed he was not. After several more hours and no sleep I requested an epidural, which unfortunately was not fully effective and alleviated pain only on the right side of my body. Every now and then my ob/gyn would pop his head in to say that if I didn't progress, I would need a c-section. Several hours later he informed me that my hips were probably too small and it was time for a c-section. I gave in! After all this time I was exhausted, defeated, and completely overwhelmed. When my son was born he was anterior facing after all, and I was informed that if he had been posterior I could have pushed him out. My postpartum period was very difficult as I did not have a good support system, had trouble with my milk supply, and overall felt depressed that I could not birth or feed my baby the right way.

Shortly after my son turned two years old, we started trying for a second baby. I was prepared to get pregnant very quickly again but was not conceiving. I started researching nutrition, but even after months of making very healthy changes I still was not pregnant. After trying for 7 months I went to see Donna Zubrod, who introduced me to the Arvigo Techniques of Maya Abdominal Therapy®.

PRACTITIONER PERSPECTIVE I have had the pleasure of working with childbearing women for several years now. When we are discussing their birth stories, I am always struck by how dramatic the differences can be in how they respond to their experiences. Given two women who experienced an identical hospital birth with multiple interventions, one woman will have a neutral reaction while the other will be left traumatized by the experience and in need of physical and emotional healing. The latter is how it was with Emma.

When I first met Emma, it was evident she was unhappy with the birth of her first son and how that process had made her feel. She came to see me with the intent to prepare for a Vaginal Birth after Caesarean (VBAC) and a more natural birth experience for her second child. She had been trying to conceive for more than half a year without success. Her periods had been light and short in duration (2 to 3 days) with thick clots at the beginning of the flow, and she was experiencing considerable discomfort around her c-section scar.

When I first examined Emma, the tissue around the c-scar was immobile; her uterus was tipped anterior and leaning toward the right side of her abdomen. Most likely, the tissue tension was causing the discomfort in her scar area, and uterine malposition was most likely the cause of reproductive concerns. The tissues in her upper and mid abdomen also felt immobile, and she shared with me that at times she felt constipated. Initially, Emma was apprehensive about the abdominal massage, but she was able to relax within a few minutes. Her low back and pelvic bones were misaligned, and the sacrum was tender. At the end of the session we discussed the importance of self-care massage. She was committed to self-care massage if it would help her to achieve a successful VBAC. In addition, she was to use castor oil packs and increase her water intake.

Two months later Emma returned, reporting her period had lengthened to 4 to 5 days, with a healthy flow and no clots. She noticed an increase in cervical mucus when ovulating that wasn't there before. She was still feeling some tightness in her lower right abdomen where she felt her uterus was still malpositioned. In applying the Arvigo techniques much had changed since our first visit as her upper abdomen was feeling more fluid and movable. The tissue in her lower abdomen remained about the same, and the pelvis was still out of alignment. A complete Arvigo session was applied. Upon reviewing how she was performing her self-care massage, I suggested she could apply more pressure.

Emma returned the following week and noted her elimination had improved; she remarked it felt more complete. The tissue in her lower abdomen was softer and more mobile as was her entire abdomen. The area around her incision line was softer as well. Posteriorly, the corrections made the previous week had held so her pelvic bones were now aligned.

As she left my office, Emma mentioned that she and her husband were going to attempt to conceive this cycle. A few weeks later she ecstatically reported that she was pregnant!

Emma's Experience

The abdominal massage was emotionally uncomfortable for me at first, but I decided to work through it. Donna explained that my immobile c-section scar tissue and uterus placement were most likely contributing to my inability to conceive. Once again my uterus was failing me, but I wanted to have another baby and committed to daily self-care massage. I have to admit initially it was a chore! I had to rub my stupid uterus because it never did anything right. I kept thinking, "This better work; my uterus better respond." Despite my negative attitude, I persevered and started feeling positive changes. The scar tissue was clearing and softening, I could feel my uterus under my hands as I did the self-care massage. It was great to hear Donna confirm the changes I was seeing when I saw her for another session. With this shift my relationship with my uterus and body was changing. When I did the self-care work, I did so with love. Sometimes I even cried when I was doing my massage; I was starting to believe in my body again. Within two months of my first session with Donna and performing daily Arvigo self-care massage I was pregnant. It was such a wonderful feeling to take control of my health and my body again.

Donna Zubrod's professional biography appears on page 53.

Preparing for a Successful Vaginal Birth after Caesarean

Fear knocked on the door.
Faith answered it, but
no one was there.

—DR. ROSITA ARVIGO

Emma (CONTINUED)   For the first 20 weeks of my pregnancy I did my own energy work above my abdomen, mimicking the Arvigo self-care massage with my hands without actually touching my body. Immediately, I felt connected with my body and baby. I knew that we were working together this time. I committed to listening to my body. This was very difficult to do while working in a fast-paced sales job and having a three-year-old. But every night I would lie quietly in bed and get in touch with my abdomen. I would close my eyes and listen to what my body was saying during that time. This was different from my first pregnancy. I did not love my body then; it was something that was just there, and I was emotionally detached from it.

I returned to see Donna for an Arvigo Therapy prenatal session when I was 20 weeks pregnant. In addition to my treatment she taught me self-care massage for pregnancy that I was to do until my baby was born. Doing the self-care massage each day was my sacred time to connect with myself and baby. My baby loved it when I would massage my belly. Mostly, he loved it when Donna would massage my belly. He would always start out quite active at the beginning of each session and would gradually fall asleep during my time with her. I was sitting quite a bit at work, which was causing me some back pain. Working with Donna was very effective at relieving all the sacrum and low back and hip pain I was having.

My sessions with Donna were very special. I knew the work we were doing physically and emotionally was setting me up for a successful labor and birth. I felt empowered and had a sense of knowing that I would give birth the way I wanted. I knew that I had everything I needed to give birth naturally.

My due date came and went (I was not surprised since I was late with my first as well). However, being a VBAC I was being monitored closely and was on the clock again as I approached week 42. I had an appointment with my midwife who had said that at this point the risks were beginning to outweigh the benefits, and I would need to be induced or have a c-section in a couple of days if labor did not start. Tears filled my eyes. We worked so hard preparing my body physically and emotionally. I could not believe this was happening. For a few hours negative thoughts ran through my head: "Your body can't give birth . . . You are not meant to have babies . . . Who are you kidding?" I just lay in bed and cried. I cried hard. I cried hard for my son that I could not give birth to, I cried for my body that I doubted, I cried that I may not have the chance to ever have a vaginal delivery, and I cried because I had worked so hard and had come so far to let it end like this. Then the crying stopped. I calmly started to rub my belly. I spoke to my baby, telling him that it was time. I had done everything I could do to prepare for this moment. I surrendered at that moment to my body. I let my mind go and let my body do what it needed to do and went to sleep. That morning I awoke to contractions. I had been having early labor signs for three weeks, so I tried not to get too excited. I went downstairs to get some water, and the contractions were not going away. They were getting closer together. I sat in a tub at home with my sister and my husband nearby.

I was managing my contractions with ease. I was not scared. I knew everything was going to be OK.

Eventually, my body told me it was time to go. We loaded up in my van and started our journey to the hospital. The contractions were intense and coming quickly. I sat hanging over the backseat in the car and watched all the lights pass by in the early morning. I remained centered and felt confident. We arrived at the hospital, and I knew we were close. They got me up to a room quickly. They checked me, and I was almost at 10 centimeters. I felt most comfortable squatting on the floor, where I stayed totally inside myself, feeling each surge but at the same time feeling safe and calm. The midwife asked me if I could feel my baby's head when I reached inside. I slowly reached down and there he was—my baby! The midwife wanted a better look, so I got up in the bed but still squatted. She looked at me and said, "You are having this baby soon, and you are doing it vaginally." I cried. The contractions were in my back, and once again I suspected he was facing anterior. When she checked, he was facing anterior so my midwife helped me into some different positions to get him to turn the right way. Soon it was time to push. This was the best part. It was like everything stopped, and the contractions did not seem to hurt at all. They were just helping me push my baby out. After only seven hours of active labor, I gave birth the way I wanted to a happy, healthy 8-pound, 3-ounce boy! It was the happiest moment of my life. I have never felt so confident and amazed by my body. I felt so good I was ready to do it all over again!

PRACTITIONER PERSPECTIVE   At 20 weeks I began the Arvigo Therapy prenatal sessions with Emma. At that time she was experiencing digestion and elimination issues. I noted her uterus was slightly off midline and leaning to the right. Posteriorly, her back muscles were tight and pelvis slightly out of alignment. She received a full Arvigo Therapy pregnancy session and was instructed in self-care massage for pregnancy.

At our next monthly session Emma reported her elimination and digestion had improved, and she felt this was because of the self care. I noticed that her uterus was no longer tilted to the right and that her pelvic bones were balanced. I continued to work with Emma regularly throughout her pregnancy. Her uterus and pelvis remained balanced, and I focused massage on her low back and gluteal muscles to relieve the discomforts of pregnancy. She continued to feel fairly relaxed during her pregnancy and reported how much she enjoyed her self-care time. It was wonderful to see her body respond to assist the baby to naturally find its optimum position for a vaginal birth.

Emma's Experience

The Arvigo work helped empower me to connect with my body and my baby. It took me on an emotional healing journey. My Arvigo Therapy prenatal sessions with Donna and the self-care massage taught me how to love and believe in my body. Once I truly let go of my previous birth experience and negative thoughts and went within my body, everything happened that needed to happen. It happened without fear, surrounded by love and a knowledge that my body can indeed birth.

Donna Zubrod's professional biography appears on page 53.

Vaginal Birth After Caesarean (VBAC) The practice of birthing a baby vaginally after a previous baby has been delivered through caesarean section is known as vaginal birth after caesarean (VBAC). A cesarean delivery can be a life-saving procedure for the mother and her child. However, it is also major abdominal surgery, putting the mother and her infant at increased risk of infections, hemorrhage, transfusions, and injury to other organs, anesthesia complications, and maternal mortality two to four times greater than that for a vaginal birth. Long-term complications in subsequent pregnancies and labors include risk for uterine rupture and placental problems. Studies also show that a caesarean delivery, particularly when it was unexpected, may put some women at increased psychological risk for depression and post-traumatic stress. The current c-section birth rate is close to 33 percent; 35 years ago it was 5 percent. Some mothers who have a c-section know before becoming pregnant again that next time they want to plan a VBAC. The rate at which VBAC is attempted today is 10 percent, falling from 26 percent in the early 1990s. According to the American Pregnancy Association, 90 percent of women who have undergone caesarean deliveries are candidates for VBAC, a safer alternative to a routine repeat cesarean. If you have a healthy pregnancy, have a low horizontal scar on the uterus and go into labor on your own at term, you have about a 70 to 75 percent chance that you and your baby will have a safe, normal birth. The American College of Obstetricians and Gynecologists recently updated its opinion on VBAC and stated, "VBAC is safer than repeat cesarean and VBAC with more than one previous cesarean does not pose any increased risk." (*Midwifery Today* , no. 36, p. 47)

Support for Postpartum Uterine Prolapse

When you really listen to
yourself, you can heal yourself.

—CEANNE DEROHAN

Sue I was 35 years old when I gave birth to my second baby following a normal pregnancy and problem-free delivery. About two weeks following this birth, I picked up my two-year-old son, who weighed about 30 pounds, and to my dismay my uterus fell out of my body! At that moment I felt a strong pressure and pulling sensation associated with difficulty walking, and this was quite painful at times. I immediately called my ob/gyn office and scheduled an appointment with Cindy Aspromonte, a nurse practitioner in the office. I knew she was a practitioner of the Arvigo Techniques of Maya Abdominal Therapy® and that the philosophy of this therapy was holistic, so I knew I was in the right place.

Cindy saw me that day, and after an examination determined that I had a significant uterine prolapse as my cervix was hanging outside of my vagina. She performed Arvigo Therapy and was able to get my uterus back in place. She instructed me to stay off my feet for several days and to avoid lifting my older child for a few days, taught me how to do self-care massage and use a faja, and recommended herbal support and tinctures.

PRACTITIONER PERSPECTIVE   Fortunately, I was able to see Sue the same day that she contacted me. As a woman's health nurse practitioner who specializes in Arvigo Therapy, I was able to perform a gynecological exam as part of my findings. When Sue told me that she thought her uterus had fallen out, I did not expect the degree of uterine prolapse that I witnessed. On her initial examination it was evident she had a uterine prolapse since the cervix and part of the uterus were outside her body. She had a stage 3 uterine prolapse, which is significant. Her cervix was out, but the entire uterus had not prolapsed (procidentia) since part of the uterus was still in the vagina and the back wall of the vagina (apex) was fairly well supported. Generally, in older postmenopausal women, it is difficult to get the uterus to stay up after such a degree of prolapse by doing Arvigo Therapy alone. However, given Sue's age, her overall good health, and excellent tissue strength, her prognosis was good. In addition, she had nutritional intake that supports health and healing.

After the initial exam I pushed the uterus into the pelvic bowl vaginally. Once it was in place, I applied the Arvigo Therapy to the lower pelvis to improve circulation to the organs and ligaments of the pelvis as well as improving lymph and nerve flow. The upper abdominal protocol was applied, and I felt a small amount of tension gently releasing. After the session, Sue felt very relaxed and had much less pelvic pressure, since her uterus was back in place. I was curious to see what would happen after she stood up. I placed a faja on her, taught her how to tie it herself next time, and asked her to stand up. Her uterus did not fall out. I was delighted!

In addition, I recommended use of a faja, herbal support, and limited lifting of anything for a few days to seeing if her uterus would remain in place. As a long-standing practitioner, in my experience the sooner these techniques are applied following a prolapse (ideally, within a day or two), the more likely they will work. My backup plan for Sue if this plan was unsuccessful was to discuss using a pessary. If a pessary was not successful, it would not bode well since many women end up having surgery to treat their prolapse if natural methods are ineffective.

She was sent home with the following instructions:

- Rest as much as possible, lying horizontal to avoid the pull of gravity when standing up
- Wear a faja when walking or standing
- Herbal support: daily nourishing tea with red raspberry leaf, nettles, oat straw, 2 to 4 cups per day
- Self-care massage daily

Sue returned for her six week postpartum exam, and her pelvic exam was completely normal. Her uterus was in perfect position and she was well rested and back to normal. She was enjoying her new baby and older child and was adjusting well. She continued to gradually increase her activities in moderation, doing all of the things we had discussed in her plan of care.

Sue's Experience
The second day after my Arvigo Therapy session I felt that my uterus remained up, and I was able to do a little more activity. I was compliant with Cindy's advice, and just took it slowly, continuing to do the Arvigo self-care massage every day and wearing the faja as much as possible. After several weeks, I did not have to use the faja as much. I continued with the self-care massage and herbal support. I'm delighted to report that my uterus stayed up and has remained in place to this day—seven years later! I feel so grateful for this experience.

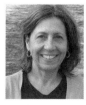

Cindy Aspromonte RN-C, NP, AHN-BC, HTCP-I   Cindy Aspromonte is a nationally recognized certified women's healthcare nurse practitioner and board-certified advanced practice holistic nurse, a Healing Touch certified practitioner and instructor, and a certified practitioner and instructor through the Arvigo Institute. She successfully integrates several different holistic modalities into her care with women, serving as a bridge by walking between the worlds of complementary and integrative medicine, traditional indigenous practices, and modern medicine. Cindy has studied with many indigenous elders of North and Central America. Cindy works at a Denver, Colorado, center for women's pelvic health.

Pelvic Organ Prolapse   The pelvic organs (uterus, vagina, bowel, bladder) are held in place by the muscles of the pelvic floor, ligaments, and layers of connective tissue called fascia. When these structures become torn, stretched, and/or weak, and can no longer provide support, the pelvic organs can drop downward, away from their optimal positions within the abdominal cavity. The primary cause of pelvic organ prolapse is childbirth. Other factors include menopause, aging, prior pelvic surgery, chronic straining. Studies show that up to 40 percent of women have some form of prolapse, with symptoms ranging from mild to severe. Symptoms may range from a feeling of heaviness, stress incontinence, or pain during sex to the organs actually bulging out of the vagina. Treatment includes lifestyle changes, weight loss, exercises, and pessaries. Some pelvic support problems may be helped by surgery, but it may not alleviate all the symptoms. Prolapse can recur after surgery. The factors that caused a woman to experience prolapse in the first place are still there and can cause it to happen again.

Relief for Unrelenting Postpartum Pain

*Who knows where inspiration
comes from. Perhaps it arises from
desperation. Perhaps it comes
from the flukes of the universe,
the kindness of the muses.*

—AMY TAN

Matilda   I was 3 months postpartum and could not sit, stand, hold, or dance with my baby without being in excruciating pain. My ob/gyn told me I probably had nerve entrapment in the scar tissue of my perineum (ouch!) and that I should see a physical therapist that specializes in the pelvic floor. Unfortunately, I would have to wait 6 to 8 weeks for that appointment. It hurt like electricity zinging me down there, and it was also psychologically difficult since I couldn't hold my baby without being in pain. It also kept me from exercising, walking outings with my moms' group, and seeing friends. A midwife I knew recommended that I consider trying the Arvigo Techniques of Maya Abdominal Therapy® and put me in touch with Abigail Reagan, who specialized in this work, and I immediately made an appointment. Someone could have told me to spread peanut butter over it down there, and I would have tried it, I was so desperate.

A few weeks later, I experienced Arvigo Therapy with Abigail. She had me fill out a very thorough intake form beforehand, and we reviewed it in detail when I met with her in person. I noted that she took a very holistic view of my health, which I appreciated. The bodywork was gentle and the table/headrest comfortable. We chatted throughout and I got the sense she had a good working knowledge of the body and how to heal it. At the end of the session she instructed me on how to do the self-care massage and apply a castor oil pack daily, and she also recommended some supplements.

PRACTITIONER PERSPECTIVE I could sense Matilda's desperation when she contacted me. She had had six postpartum appointments with her ob/gyn because of the slow healing of her perineal tear after the long labor with her first child. Despite cauterization of granulation tissue with silver nitrate by her doctor at four weeks postpartum, using lidocaine cream, and taking Motrin daily, she was still in pain by nine weeks postpartum.

Matilda seemed skeptical as to how Arvigo Therapy would be able to help her when her ob/gyn was not able to offer any solution other than an explanation that her pain might be caused by pudendal nerve entrapment that would go away in a few more months. In her online research, Matilda had found that all pudendal nerve pain is chronic. She described her pain as "intense and sharp" and said it felt worse on her left side than on the right. She shared that she had tried massage, craniosacral therapy, and chiropractic in the weeks since the birth, but nothing had relieved her pain.

During my assessment I found Matilda's uterus to be anteflexed to the left, her upper abdomen very tight and tender, lymph congestion in the left inguinal area, pelvic bones misaligned and her sacrum restricted in its movement. Interestingly, there was no tenderness around her coccyx or ischium. I was a bit surprised that there was no pain around this area since I knew the pudendal nerve travels through here. Matilda seemed to enjoy the treatment, and got off the table more relaxed. She was disappointed (and so was I) that her pain was not immediately improved.

I taught Matilda how to do an easy self-care massage and advised her to perform it for 5 minutes daily. I also recommended that she wear cloth menstrual pads saturated with castor oil every day to help soften and heal her perineal tissue. She was having a lot of anxiety about life, finances, and the future, which was exacerbated by dealing with daily pain so I suggested a bottle of Nerve Tonic, one of the Rainforest Remedies, and she accepted it. Finally, we discussed a few dietary changes and supplements to help with inflammation (eliminate gluten; take bromelain and vitamin D).

When Matilda left my office I could tell that she was discouraged that she hadn't had relief from her pain and that she thought I was just another one of a long list of things she'd tried for her situation. I had faith, though, that she would have a shift, because in my experience it can take some time for symptoms to improve with natural healing methods. Occasionally, clients even find symptoms worsen for a day or two before significant improvement.

Matilda's Experience
I followed Abigail's instructions and literally the next day I woke up and felt noticeably better, 80 to 90 percent better, in fact. I was stunned. I had feared I would live with this pain for years. I still had discomfort, but I was so happy to be out of extreme pain after so long. I met with Abigail for two more follow-up Arvigo Therapy sessions over the next 2 months and to receive her health/nutrition/healing advice. I was also finally able to get an appointment and work with a pelvic floor physical therapist during most of this time. By my second session with Abigail I was fully relieved of pain and able to do all the activities a busy new mom needs to do.

I am very impressed with how knowledgeable Arvigo Therapists are about health and healing. They understand the body very well. Abigail changed my life and added to my knowledge of health and healing.

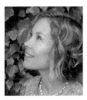

Abigail Reagan LM, CPM (www.rebirthmidwifery.com) Abigail is a California licensed midwife and certified professional midwife who has been supporting women and families in the San Francisco area since 1993. Her passion to guide women healthily through the childbearing year—especially in preparation for labor—led Abigail to study the Arvigo Techniques of Maya Abdominal Therapy®. In her years of working closely with women, she came to understand and trust that our bodies have innate wisdom and an ability to come into homeostasis, or balance, when supplied with the foods, nutrients, and supportive therapies they need. As a certified Arvigo practitioner, Abigail works with women at all stages in their lives to optimize healthy menses, fertility, pregnancy, menopause, digestion, and more. She is a certified Arvigo Self Care teacher and assists Rosita Arvigo in teaching the Advanced Pregnancy class.

Male Reproductive Conditions

Becoming Symptom Free from Chronic Pelvic Pain and Benign Prostatic Hyperplasia

Choose to be optimistic.
It feels better.

—DALAI LAMA XIV

John I was 63 when I first met Karl Monahan. My physio referred me to him because she felt his more holistic approach to pelvic pain may be more suitable to my condition. For 2 years I had been suffering with chronic prostatitis, also known as chronic pelvic pain syndrome (CPPS). I was also diagnosed with benign prostatic hyperplasia (BPH) 7 years ago. At the time when my symptoms started, I was going through a divorce and my daughter was suffering with her obsessive compulsive disorder. I was getting more and more anxious about both situations and felt that they were completely out of my control. I have suffered with irritable bowel syndrome (IBS) in the past and it was making a bit of a comeback to top things off. I was struggling to sit down for any length of time and being an economics tutor this was not great. Walking for greater distances was becoming an issue and standing was also painful. My symptoms included lower back pain, pain in my perineum and base of penis. My prostate pain felt like I was sitting on a golf ball! In addition, there were times when there was pain in my lower abdomen, especially around the pubic bone, with discomfort in the inner thighs. I was also experiencing problems achieving orgasm.

119

My physio felt I had weakened gluteus and groin muscles, which was causing all of my symptoms. My urologist had prescribed medications for the BPH and for general pain. I just felt stuck as nothing was improving, the quality of my life was decreasing, and I was fed up with the way I was feeling. I was in good health, I exercised regularly (albeit slightly less since having the pelvic pain), I ate sensibly, and I didn't drink or smoke, so why was all this happening to me?

PRACTITIONER PERSPECTIVE   John was amongst the first handful of patients I had seen suffering with chronic prostatitis or CPPS. He was a little anxious about what to expect and how Arvigo Therapy would affect his symptoms. He certainly didn't want his symptoms to worsen.

During the initial session, I checked to see if my findings were consistent with what the physio was reporting. John exhibited imbalances in range of motion in major muscle groups around his pelvis; for example his left quadriceps were tighter than the right, his hamstrings were tighter on the right side and his adductors or inner thighs were tighter on the right side as well. He had more tenderness in his lower left back. His lower abdomen was tighter than his upper. I also noted that he had a pattern of tenderness and fibrotic tissues around the left side of his sacrum and coccyx.

At the end of the session, I suggested a number of stretches for his major leg muscle groups (quadriceps, hamstrings, adductors, hip flexors, and gluteus muscles) to address some of the imbalances he was experiencing. We discussed his diet, and I gave him a healthy diet sheet to help guide him with his meal plans to reduce refined sugar intake and sugar cravings in what was otherwise a well-balanced diet. I felt that if he was suffering from IBS, this may trigger further inflammation in the pelvic regions and further aggravate his prostatitis. In addition, I recommended he apply hot and cold compresses to his perineum in 5-minute increments to help increase lymphatic flow and reduce any inflammation to this hard-to-reach area. He was instructed in home self-care massage as well and was adamant he would be vigilant with his homework.

Three weeks later John returned for his follow-up appointment delighted with his progress as he found significant relief in all of his symptoms. His commitment to his self-care massage and other homework suggestions was exactly what I would ask for in a patient, focusing on all of the areas we advised with great care and attention.

The pain in his prostate was still the most dominant of all his symptoms, but the other areas of pain had all reduced to 1s and 2s on a scale of 10, with 10 being the most painful and 0 being no pain at all. John had been able to balance those major muscle groups in his legs and hips with only his right quadriceps still holding a little tension compared to his right side.

Overall, his symptoms had significantly reduced, and I was very pleased with his progress. We stayed in contact via e-mail for a number of months to monitor his progress and to allow for any guidance should he require it. He attended a number of my Prostatitis Support Group meetings where he let me know that he was experiencing a slight increase in perineum and scrotal pain from sitting for long periods as well as increased urinary frequency. This was often due to external stressful situations, but I assured him that if he kept on top of his self-care massage, stretches, daily exercise routine, and healthy diet, he would be able to manage these symptoms and reduce them significantly.

John's Experience

It is now 20 months since my initial appointment with Karl. My symptoms are almost completely gone. I continued to work with Karl here and there so he could check that nothing else was affecting my improvement rate. I also had an MRI to ensure there were no soft tissue concerns, and the results came back clear. I was happy when Karl confirmed for me that apart from some minimal general tension in the abdominal and pelvic region, I seemed to be in good shape.

I have started having cognitive behavioural therapy sessions to help me so that I don't worry about the future so much. I am increasingly more confident that as long as I continue with my healthy lifestyle routine and self-care massage I will remain pain and symptom free.

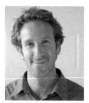 **Karl Monahan** (www.thebodyworkspractice.co.uk)   Karl qualified as a registered massage therapist in London, England, in 2001. He has since continued his evolution to become a sports and pelvic pain therapist. Karl was the first man to offer the highly specialised Arvigo Techniques of Maya Abdominal Therapy® in Europe, and is one of a growing team of Arvigo therapists in the UK. He lectured at the Biannual Arvigo Therapy Convention in Mexico in 2011 on the benefits of Arvigo Therapy in treating male chronic pelvic pain syndrome and prostatitis, one of his areas of speciality. He currently teaches sports massage, remedial massage, sports and exercise nutrition, and corrective exercise at North East Surrey College of Technology. He plans to complete his Arvigo Therapy teaching qualification within the next few years. Karl is the co-director, founder, and head therapist at The Bodyworks Practice, Surrey, England.

Chronic Prostatitis/Chronic Pelvic Pain Syndrome (CP/CPPS)   Pelvic or perineal pain without evidence of urinary tract infection and lasting longer than 3 months is diagnosed as chronic prostatitis/chronic pelvic pain syndrome (CP/CPPS). Symptoms may wax and wane. Pain can range from mild to debilitating. Pain may radiate to the back and rectum, making sitting uncomfortable. Pain can be present in the perineum, testicles, tip of penis, pubic area, or bladder area. Unexplained fatigue, abdominal pain, constant burning pain in the penis, and urinary frequency may also be present. Frequent urination and increased urgency may suggest interstitial cystitis (inflammation centered in bladder rather than prostate). Post-ejaculatory pain is a hallmark of this condition and serves to distinguish CP/CPPS patients from men with BPH. Some men report low libido, sexual dysfunction, and erectile difficulties. The symptoms of CP/CPPS appear to result from interplay between psychological factors and dysfunction in the immune, neurological, and endocrine systems. There are no definitive diagnostic tests for CP/CPPS. This is a poorly understood disorder, even though it accounts for 90 to 95 percent of prostatitis diagnoses. It is found in men of any age, with the peak incidence in men aged 35 to 45 years, with the overall prevalence of symptoms in 6.3 percent of the male population. New evidence suggests that the prevalence of CP/CPPS is much higher in teenage males than once suspected. Treatment is often a combination of medication (antidepressants and anti-anxiety), psychological therapy (including progressive relaxation techniques), and physical therapy focusing on pelvic floor relaxation (trigger point release, yoga). Biofeedback physical therapy to relearn how to control pelvic floor muscles may also be useful.

Taking Charge to Self Manage Benign Prostate Hyperplasia

There is no magic wand that can resolve our problems.
The solution rests with our work and discipline.

—JOSE EDUARDO DOS SANTOS

Cliff I feel like the list of medications my doctor suggests as I age keeps getting longer and longer. I know that with those medications come side effects, and I really want to minimize the amount of medications I am taking. I'm 50 pounds overweight, 55 years old, and have had pain in every joint from the waist down since childhood. I try to stay active even with the pain to keep my weight under control. My biggest concern of late is BPH (benign prostatic hyperplasia) with a slowly climbing PSA (prostate-specific antigen) and related erectile dysfunction. I was using medications to help me have a normal urinary stream as well as erectile dysfunction medication. My chiropractor referred me to Michelle Rankin for Arvigo Therapy.

I had no idea what to expect, but Michelle put me at ease. After the session she instructed me in home self-care massage and recommended drinking corn silk tea and doing exercises to rebalance my pelvis. Within 2 months of performing self-care massage on a routine basis I was able to stop the medication for urinary flow and decreased the erectile dysfunction medication by about 50 percent.

I am pleased to report my urinary stream is as good if not better by doing the self-care massage than it was when I was taking the medication!

PRACTITIONER PERSPECTIVE   The chiropractor who referred Cliff to me generally sends me clients with complicated medical histories and Cliff was no different. He presented with pain in his neck, lumbar spine, both hips and both knees, with worse pain on the right and worse with rest. He takes two prescriptions for high blood pressure, urinary flow problems, and erectile dysfunction. He had a total hip replacement on the left in 2009, hernia repair with mesh in his lower left abdomen, and a repaired varicocele in 1995. He was especially concerned about BPH with his steadily climbing PSA and erectile dysfunction and came to me specifically in hopes that both problems could be treated without medication.

He reported his right leg was shorter than his left during childhood. Following his hip replacement, his left leg now measured a half inch longer than his right. Assessing him during the Arvigo Therapy session, I noted his pelvic alignment was fairly normal though his low back, hip, and gluteal muscles were in spasm, and he had trouble sitting on hard surfaces. His sacrum and coccyx were immobile and painful. Due to a hernia repair he had done previously, I modified the lower abdominal massage so as not to disrupt the mesh that was supporting the hernia repair. After the session he noted immediate relief from the discomfort. I taught him core-strengthening exercises to decrease the muscle spasms and to relax and assist his pelvis to maintain alignment. I also instructed him in self-care massage and gave him some corn silk tea to brew at home.

Cliff returned to my office 6 weeks later and reported that due to his daily commitment to self-care massage he discontinued the medication for urinary flow issues and decreased the erectile dysfunction medication in half.

Cliff's Experience   After 3 months of treatment I had a setback. This occurred at the time I slacked off on my home self-care massage. I began having pain in my right testicle and was diagnosed with prostatitis. My doctor suggested I restart the urinary flow medication. At the same time I recommitted to home self-care massage and another round of corn silk tea. A month later I was off the medication without further problems.

I continued to follow up with Michelle once a month for the next 6 months for additional work on my lower back and hips and by the end of that time I was sleeping twice as long at night thanks to less frequent urination and decreased pain.

I have come to realize that my options are pretty straight-forward. I can spend 8 minutes a day and perform the self-care massage Michelle taught me and check in with her regularly, or I can choose to take medications. My goal was to minimize the amount of medications I'm taking so the choice is easy for me.

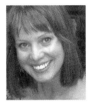

Michelle Rankin BS, LMP (www.risingmoonmassage.com) Michelle Rankin is a nationally certified Washington state massage therapist and certified Avigo Therapy practitioner, specializing in chronic pain and reproductive and digestive issues. The Arvigo Techniques of Maya Abdominal Therapy® are paramount to her treatment approach for cases of low back and hip pain as well as all reproductive and digestive issues. She uses a multifaceted approach to tackling cases of chronic pain and reproductive issues, based on her massage training and degree in exercise science.

Benign Prostatic Hyperplasia (BPH) Non-malignant enlargement of the prostate gland is known as benign prostatic hyperplasia (BPH). It generally begins when a man is in his 30s, evolves slowly, and most commonly causes symptoms only after age 50. An estimated 50 percent of men have BPH by age 50 and 75 percent by age 80; in 40 to 50 percent of these men, BPH becomes clinically significant. As the prostate gland grows in size, it compresses the urethra, which courses through the center of the prostate, impeding the flow of urine from the bladder through the urethra to the outside. It can cause urine to back up in the bladder (retention), leading to the need to urinate frequently during the day and night. Other common symptoms include a slow flow of urine, the need to urinate urgently, and difficulty starting the urinary stream. More serious problems include urinary tract infections and complete blockage of the urethra, which may be a medical emergency and can lead to kidney injury. Treatment of BPH is usually reserved for men with significant symptoms. Watchful waiting to see if the condition gets worse with medical monitoring once a year is the first line of treatment. For men with significant symptoms, medications are prescribed that carry side effects, mostly related to sexual function. For men who have not responded well to medication or those who have more severe symptoms, such as a complete inability to urinate, prostate surgery is viewed as offering the most benefits for BPH but unfortunately carries the most risks.

A Non-Pharmaceutical Solution for Erectile Dysfunction and Urinary Problems

If a man would move the world,
he must first move himself.

—SOCRATES

Dan It seems like with age I've been experiencing any man's worst fears when it comes to bedroom performance. For years I've been living with psoriasis and psoriatic arthritis as well as a chronic kidney disease. I was diagnosed with type 2 diabetes and high blood pressure a few years ago and right around the same time I started to experience frequent urination with low flow, incomplete voiding, and although I was able to orgasm, I could no longer maintain an erection. I'm only 53 and happily married so I wasn't willing to throw in the towel in the bedroom department yet. I was having chronic pain in my hips.

My son had been raving about a treatment Michelle Rankin offered named Arvigo Therapy that had helped his low back and hip pain and discreetly left one of her cards on my desk one day. Her card advertised "balancing reproductive and digestive systems" so I gave her a call.

After the session I noticed right away that my low back and hip felt much better. I hadn't even realized I had issues with back pain until she treated it. Michelle sent me home with instructions to perform self-care massage daily but life got in the way and I managed to do it only 3 days a week.

PRACTITIONER PERSPECTIVE   Dan came to me on his son's referral with quite a few chronic medical diagnoses from his health care provider. The most irritating issues for him, and the reason he came to see me, were the frequent urination and erectile dysfunction, both of which his doctors told him were just part of aging and the best they could do was offer more medications to offset the side effects of the drugs he was already taking. He was skeptical about Arvigo Therapy but hopeful that I could help.

Dan presented with spasm in his left low back and bilateral gluteal muscles. His pelvic bones were out of balance. He also had rectus diastasis which is medial vertical separation of the rectus abdominus muscle so I had to modify some of the Arvigo Therapy techniques accordingly.

He returned for his second visit two weeks later and admitted he had been performing his self-care massage only 3 days a week while standing up in the shower (it's supposed to be done while lying down). He was disappointed that he hadn't noticed any improvements yet but returned because his hip felt much better. Dan's complicated medical history did not allow me to suggest a strong herbal tincture but I urged him to give the self-care massage a chance and perform it daily. I also sent him home with corn silk tea, which is an herbal preparation known to support the urinary system for men and women.

Dan's Experience
After my second visit I started to perform the self-care massage daily and I drank the tea, which tasted exactly like boiled corn water, and I immediately noticed both more flow control during urination and my ejaculate becoming much less viscous.

I saw Michelle again for a third and final session and let her know I was absolutely thrilled with the self-care massage and the herbal tea. My bladder symptoms improved immediately once I started drinking the corn silk tea; I had much more control of the flow and less urgency and frequency. I felt that the self-care massage was making a big difference in my ability to achieve and maintain an erection. I also noticed that my ejaculate had changed from a thick cream to a thin liquid that reminded me of what I produced back in my 20s. I'm thrilled that things are moving in the right direction after only three visits, and I've pledged to continue my self care on a daily basis.

Michelle Rankin's professional biography appears on page 125.

Regaining Self-Esteem while Learning to Manage Pelvic Pain

Every patient carries his or her own doctor inside.

—ALBERT SCHWEITZER

Peter   I'm in my early 40s and for the past year I've been suffering with a number of abdominal and pelvic complaints. I'm unsure of what truly brought them on, but I'm very concerned I may have contracted a sexually transmitted disease from a previous partner. She reassures me that there is nothing to be worried about and that she is clean, yet it still does not settle my worries and concerns.

My symptoms are many: sharp burning down the urethra on urination, lower abdominal pain, pain in the perineum, a constant dull ache in the tip of the penis, pain on ejaculation, pain/pressure in the bladder with having to urinate every 20 minutes.

I have made a number of visits to the GUM (sexual health) clinic to be sure that I hadn't picked anything up; at each visit I am told that there is nothing wrong with me. I have seen my doctor a handful of times over the year, requesting further tests and scans to be carried out, each of which has been negative. My doctor has tried me on numerous antibiotics and antidepressants with very little, if any, positive effect. I have visited specialist after specialist, always being dismissed as having nothing wrong with me. This only fuels my anxieties and worries further, leaving me in a very low, desperate place.

>After a recent sexual encounter I developed a small blister from a burst blood vessel on my penis and this was ruining my life. I was desperate. A family friend told me about Karl Monahan's practice.

PRACTITIONER PERSPECTIVE   Peter was not in a good place when he came to see me, suffering from low self-esteem and a real lack of faith in the medical world. He was trying to stay on top of things, eating healthy and having some basic exercise routine. However, on really bad days he would just eat junk food and not do anything. The fact that he had to urinate every 20 minutes was not helping him stay active.

His first Arvigo Therapy session was very much about empowering Peter, helping to give him a sense of having more control over his life again. Due to his high number of visits to the GUM clinic, I was confident that he hadn't contracted anything untoward and was happy to treat as normal. Peter was a fit young man with very little tension in his body apart from his upper abdomen. I felt the upper abdominal tension was restricting his breathing, resulting in short and sharp upper lung breaths, not very conducive for allowing a relaxed state within the body. His pelvic bones were misaligned although nothing too significant when measured against other patients. He had a little tenderness around the coccyx, or tailbone, again on the right.

Peter enjoyed the session and felt that the different pressures to the back, legs, pelvis, and abdomen were very therapeutic. I gave him a stretch routine for his legs to keep him mobile and active. I suggested looking at his posture and to try deep breathing exercises to help him relax. I gave him a healthy diet sheet and told him to try and focus on what he was putting into his body. Bad food can make you feel bad; good, healthy, nutritious food will fuel your body more effectively and not give you highs and lows like junk food can. I wanted to keep things realistic and within reach for the first session. I didn't want Peter to waver from his goal. I also suggested that it would be worth investigating CBT (cognitive behavioural therapy) to help address his mind chatter and make him less worried and anxious.

Peter's second visit brought very good news: His penis blemish had been given the all-clear by the dermatologist, and he was feeling much more in control of things. He was very pleased with his own progress, sticking to his routine, which helped give him a sense of worth and something positive to focus on. He said he felt amazing for days after the last session and was keen to progress with the recommendations for home-care techniques. I recognized this as a vital turning point for Peter and for me as his Arvigo therapist. Sometimes giving too much to a patient to do can be detrimental, sometimes too little and they don't follow our suggestions; it has to be a fine balance.

Peter's urinary pain and burning were down to a minimum, as was the post-ejaculation pain. He still had increased urinary frequency, but this was not causing pain; it was more of an annoyance. Peter was also experiencing a little dribbling after urination. I was confident that moving forward and teaching him his self-care massage would help to improve both of these symptoms. Other things to note at this session were a slight discomfort in the right inguinal canal (groin/crease of the leg where it meets the body) and a little discomfort along the left side of the shaft of his penis. During the treatment I noted that the tension in his abdomen was less so (also something I felt would be managed by teaching him his self-care massage), with only a small amount of muscular tightness near his belly button. He was more aware of his posture and breathing, and his hips felt more balanced or even. His coccyx (tailbone) was still a little tender to touch.

I asked Peter to really make an effort to be more vigilant with his diet, increase his stretch regime, and resume yoga (something he used to do before he got his symptoms). I also taught Peter his self-care massage and the importance of sitz baths; hot and cold baths using Epsom salts to help ease muscular tension. At this point I felt Peter was confident with my approach and wanted to do his utmost to help himself.

Peter's third and final visit to me came roughly 2.5 months after his initial one. He felt "amazing" and was very pleased with his progress. I was thrilled for him, and he was like a different person. We spoke about what he was going to do in the New Year (it was 23rd December), how he was focused on starting up his own personal training business and had applied for a job in central London within a gym. His urinary frequency had reduced significantly, he was no longer worried about his urination, and he had a minimal amount of dribbling. His pain and burning were at a minimum, the pain he had in his right inguinal region had gone, and he had no discomfort in the shaft of his penis! He still had a small amount of tension/discomfort in his abdomen but was otherwise in very good shape.

Peter's Experience

Ever since Karl showed me how to do self-care massage, I have been doing it religiously every day. I also take regular hot and cold baths/showers, paying particular attention to my pelvis, abdomen, and groin. I have worked to build up a solid stretch and yoga routine, and I feel like I have my life back. Karl and I touch base every once in a while; it helps me to stick to my routines. I sometimes experience flare-ups of my symptoms during periods of extreme stress or when I feel run down, but I now have the tools with which to manage and reduce my symptoms. My personal training business is doing well, and I feel more in control of my life again.

Karl Monahan's professional biography appears on page 122.

Digestive Disorders and Post-Surgical Recovery

Acknowledging Stress as a
First Step in Confronting Colitis

Every day brings a choice: to
practice stress or to practice peace.
—JOAN BORYSENKO

Sandra It has been a very unpleasant and difficult experience trying
to find solutions to my chronic ulcerative colitis. Over the years I
have been sent from doctor to specialist numerous times utilizing
most of my finances and energy with no remedy. I am 27, married,
with two children under the age of four. Although I have been taking
medications and made changes to my diet, colitis flare-ups were still
occurring around times of stressful situations. At those times blood
would appear in my stools. Some of my stressors included being a new
mom, issues in my marriage, and the sudden death of my mom last
year. I also consider myself a worrier and have experienced depression
since childhood. My mother had mental health issues and abused
alcohol.

Out of frustration I found myself seeking more natural therapy
approaches to my ulcerative colitis, thinking, "What do I have to
lose?" This led me to Alex Jackson, a local practitioner of the Arvigo
Techniques of Maya Abdominal Therapy®.

PRACTITIONER PERSPECTIVE   Before starting Sandra's Arvigo Therapy session, I spent time talking with her regarding her body's response to stress and the
pain she was experiencing with colitis flare-ups. This was the first time anyone

had explained to her the connection between emotional and physical issues; she was so relieved to hear this! As I proceeded with the treatment, I noticed just how sensitive her colon was, with the descending colon tight and sensitive to touch. With gentle and slow massage Sandra began to shed a few tears, speaking of a memory of her mother with a wave of sadness coming over her while at the same time she described a sensation that her colon had softened. It was as if her colon had finally been given permission to take a breath and release what it had been storing. There were a few other tender spots in her belly, the right side of the navel and just inferior to her sternum in the solar plexus.

The abdominal massage slowly began to loosen tight areas, decreasing tissue congestion and improving organ alignment and overall circulation to the tissues. In the middle of the session Sandra stated she felt tingling in her arms and legs, and I explained to her this was due to increased circulation in her body brought about by the treatment. By the time the session was done, her abdomen felt much softer, with more tissue mobility, her spirit was lighter, and her breathing was deeper and more relaxed.

Before Sandra left, I explained to her that I have worked with many people with this condition and it seems to me that there is a connection between a stressful environment in childhood and digestive issues as an adult. Often adults with colitis store emotions and stress in the abdomen and have a difficult time expressing these emotions. In addition to the Arvigo Therapy, I recommended dietary changes, daily home self-care massage, and therapeutic counseling sessions to address her history of trauma.

Sandra's Experience

Alex called me a week later to check in on me. I told him my abdomen was a bit tender for a few days, but, overall, after just one week my symptoms had improved 80 percent, and there was no longer any blood in my stool. Alex and I are confident that my condition will continue to improve if I continue to remain diligent with my daily self-care massage. I have gained a new awareness of how stress can trigger outbreaks of colitis. Finally, after many years of being ill, I feel that I am empowered to take actions to improve my health.

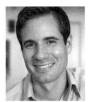

Alex Jackson LMT, NCTMB (www.centeredspirit.com)   Alex is a holistic health practitioner, specializing in Maya traditional healing methods and certified in the Arvigo Techniques of Maya Abdominal Therapy®. For the last decade, Alex's primary focus in his practice has been on traditional ways to heal the body and spirit through the abdomen. Proper balance in the core can resolve many physical ailments and emotional traumas. Alex is founder/owner of Centered Spirit, LLC, a clinic in Kansas City, Missouri, that specializes in abdominal health, therapeutic massage, and traditional healing. He treats many women with menstrual/reproductive issues such as painful periods, irregular cycles, tipped uterus, infertility, bladder pain, and more. He is also known for helping men and women with digestive problems.

Colitis   Associated with diarrhea, abdominal pain, bloating, and blood in the stool, colitis is inflammation of the inner lining of the colon. This inflammation may be due to a variety of reasons, including infection (virus, bacteria, parasite), inflammatory bowel disease (ulcerative colitis, Crohn's disease), and loss of blood supply to the colon (low blood pressure, anemia, hernia, narrowing of the supplying arteries). While many causes of colon inflammation can be treated with diet and observation, it is important to determine why inflammation has occurred because of the potential for a more serious diagnosis. Treatment of colitis often is supportive and is aimed at maintaining adequate hydration and pain control while a diagnosis is being pursued.

Finding Relief after Years of IBS Symptoms

The brain and the gastrointestinal system are so intimately connected that they should be viewed as one system, not two. When the gut acts up for no obvious physical or infectious cause, trying to heal it without considering the impact of stress and emotion is like trying to improve an employee's performance without considering his or her manager and work environment.

—LAWRENCE FRIEDMAN, MD

Kati As a licensed professional counselor I felt I was a good health care advocate for my longstanding IBS (irritable bowel syndrome), which I have suffered from for the past 18 years. I am an otherwise healthy 44-year-old woman who, for the most part, takes a natural approach to health care, but the symptoms of IBS were bothersome. For me, these were gas, abdominal bloating, and constipation, sometimes aggravated by stress and other times by diet. I wasn't taking any medications for these symptoms. I had two abdominal surgeries, one for a caesarean section for the birth of my son when I was 34 and a procedure to inflate my bladder when I was five years old for frequent urinary tract infections.

My unrelenting symptoms and preference for natural wellness solutions led me to Alex Jackson, a local practitioner of the Arvigo Techniques of Maya Abdominal Therapy®.

PRACTITIONER PERSPECTIVE   Kati's Arvigo Therapy session began with a castor oil pack on her abdomen to help with any congestion and to soften the abdominal tissues before the treatment. Beginning in the upper abdomen, I gently applied the massage techniques to help release tension in her diaphragm. Based on how the tissues were feeling, I sensed there was considerable congestion around her liver. As I continued to massage this area she reported feeling slightly nauseous, which subsided as she focused on her breath. At this time she became aware of an emotional experience, which she relayed to me in her words as "stored anger and frustration." I reassured her that this was not a coincidence as the emotion of the liver is anger. Kati went on to recall tension in her home as a child when her parents would argue, and she would develop stomach pains after witnessing the conflict. It was amazing. Almost as soon as she remembered her childhood connection with her IBS symptoms and was able feel the emotion and release it—her body changed instantly! Her breathing was much easier and relaxed, and her entire abdomen felt soft. I continued with the rest of her treatment, instructed her in self-care massage, and recommended she apply some castor oil packs to her abdomen at home.

Kati's Experience

Two weeks later I returned to see Alex and felt so much better. Imagine not having any IBS pain or constipation after the first session. It was amazing to me to think that after all these years of discomfort I had 2 weeks symptom free! I have been doing my self-care massage at home consistently and thoroughly enjoying it especially after a stressful day at work. Alex gave me another Arvigo Therapy session and I was amazed at how much deeper he was able to work in my tissues compared to my first session. My abdomen didn't feel as tense as it had the first time. I now have a deeper appreciation of the impact of stress on the body and my long-term struggle with this condition. I understand that my body's reaction to stress is to protect and tighten, especially in my gut. I now have the tools of my own hands to help manage and remedy my condition. Thank you, Arvigo Therapy!

Alex Jackson's professional biography appears on page 139.

Irritable Bowel Syndrome (IBS)   A disorder that leads to abdominal pain and cramping, changes in bowel movements, and other symptoms is known as irritable bowel syndrome (IBS). It is not clear why people develop IBS: There is a variety of triggers. Since the intestine is connected to the brain, bowel function nerves can become more active during stress, causing the intestines to be more sensitive and squeeze (contract) more. IBS can occur at any age, but it often begins in the teen years or early adulthood. It is one of the most common disorders seen by doctors, as high as 20 percent, and twice as common in women as in men. The main symptoms of IBS are abdominal pain, fullness, gas, and bloating that have been present for at least 3 days a month for the last 3 months. Symptoms vary from person to person and range from mild to severe, with most people having mild symptoms. Some people may switch between constipation and diarrhea, or mostly have one or the other. For others, symptoms may get worse for a few weeks or a month, and then decrease for a while, or be present most of the time. There is no test to diagnose IBS but tests may be done to rule out other problems. The goal of treatment is symptom reduction through lifestyle (exercise, more sleep) and dietary changes; however, no specific diet can be recommended for IBS as the condition differs from person to person. Medications are also prescribed to treat the symptoms, and therapy may help in cases of anxiety and/or depression. Irritable bowel syndrome may be a lifelong condition. For some people, symptoms are disabling and reduce the ability to work, travel, and attend social events.

Managing Chronic Constipation
and Bowel Obstruction:
An Integrative Approach

Be faithful in small things
because it is in them that
your strength lies.

—MOTHER TERESA

Mara   I am a married woman in my late 30s with one child. I have had long-standing issues with constipation (stools are hard to pass and infrequent; I need to strain; bowel evacuation feels incomplete; stools are hard and small).

In 1986 I had an appendectomy, causing a lot of bowel adhesions after the surgery. Thirteen years later in 2009 emergency surgery was required due to bowel obstruction from these adhesions. I had a full recovery from that surgery, but within 3 months bowel adhesions re-developed, requiring a second surgery in 2010 to remove these adhesions that were obstructing the bowel. Prior to both of these bowel obstruction surgeries, I was in extreme pain, experienced a lot of nausea. Post-surgery recovery required a long time.

At my initial session, Jennifer O'Hagan explained how the Arvigo Techniques of Maya Abdominal Therapy® may help to improve my health issues and showed me a very simple massage on my abdomen. She also talked about the benefits of castor oil packs. I found these suggestions easy to learn and to do and have been very consistent with doing my daily self-care massage and castor oil packs.

PRACTITIONER PERSPECTIVE   When I first met Mara it was about 6 weeks after her 2010 abdominal surgery. It was apparent that she and her husband were both very frightened by the bowel obstructions in the past, and wanted to find a way of preventing their recurrence. Stress levels were very high due to the pain of her past experiences, and she was afraid she would not live through the next time or another surgery. During our intake discussion I also found out that she regularly has painful periods with severe cramping.

Mara's surgical sites were still in the process of healing and there was a lot of congestion/fluid along the incision site and on the right side of her abdomen. Her abdomen was painful to the touch. She could not lie on her stomach. Her sacrum and left hip were very sore and tender to the touch. She had a large central scar that went from her sternum to below her umbilicus as well as a large scar on her lower right abdomen.

At her first session I applied the treatment with very light pressure due to her discomfort and the state of the scars. She was taught the self-care massage. I emphasized that she was to do this daily, using feather-light strokes, and to apply castor oil packs to her abdomen daily, taking a break on weekends. In addition, we discussed the importance of improving her water intake, dietary changes such as dried fruits soaked in water, and food combining to decrease gas and bloating. We reviewed her supplements and made some additional suggestions for B vitamins and digestive enzymes and recommended applying calendula ointment to her scars to promote healing. Finally, we discussed the importance of walking 20 to 30 minutes every day and getting more sleep.

Mara returned for a second treatment about 2 weeks later, reporting she was implementing all of my recommendations and noticing a decrease in bloating and the gassy feeling. The knots in her stomach were not present; bowel movements had improved. The abdominal incisions appeared healed but were still sensitive to touch, so only light pressure was applied at this session. She was unable to lie on her stomach and received the posterior protocol in a side-lying position. She was to continue the same home care plan as we discussed at her first visit. The dietary changes didn't improve her symptoms significantly, so I recommended she be tested for gluten intolerance/sensitivity as gluten can cause inflammation in the gut and could be contributing to the blockages.

In two weeks Mara returned for her third visit. The incision was sufficiently healed and less tender, so I could apply the techniques with more pressure, and I encouraged her to do the same with her own self-care massage at home. Instead of the fiber supplement she was taking, I recommended she switch to slippery elm bark powder tea since it is a mucilaginous fiber which is known to assist healing of the mucosal lining as well as supporting bowel function. Although she has still not been tested for gluten tolerance she has been decreasing her gluten intake.

At her next visit, Mara reported that her bowels and bloating were much better. Her abdominal pain was so much less that she could now lie on her stomach. Cramping with her period was significantly less. Mara felt the slippery elm bark tea was helping her stools be more regular and well-formed. She noted that whenever she goes out with her girlfriends for dinner, her symptoms worsen that night and for several days after, but if she eats what she prepares at home she does much better. We talked again about foods that tend to cause inflammation (gluten, dairy, soy, corn, sugar/high fructose corn syrup/artificial sweeteners, eggs) and that she should try to reduce/avoid them as her symptoms do improve when they are eliminated from her diet. Mara is still very stressed due to issues with her daughter, frustrated with still feeling like she's recovering and wishing she could do more, and having trouble sleeping. I recommended drinking teas of lemon balm, chamomile, or linden throughout the day and in evening; powering down her computer by 7 p.m.; trying a lavender/hops sleep pillow; and taking white chestnut flower essence before bed if she's having trouble "turning her head off." Her digestion seems to be improved so I recommended stopping the digestive enzymes with meals and taking them between meals, and also adding one digestive enzyme to her castor oil when doing a pack.

The next time I worked with Mara she had just come back from vacation. While she was away, she found it difficult to follow her self-care activities, and her diet consisted of a lot of processed foods, gluten, and dairy. Many of her symptoms returned; she had a lot of discomfort, bloating, and constipation. I recommended she resume her self care. When we spoke a few weeks later over the phone, Mara was back on track with her diet, self-care massage, and castor oil packs and feeling fine.

Mara's Experience My symptoms started to improve after my initial Arvigo Therapy session with Jen. I have found that with diet changes, daily self-care massage, and castor oil packs, I am able to maintain good digestion and elimination. My scars seem less ropy when I touch them, and my abdomen feels softer. Bloating is much less as long as long as I pay attention to my diet and food combinations. Cramping during my period is barely noticeable. It has been 3 years since I first went to see Jen, and I have had no recurrence of bowel obstruction.

Integrating the self-care techniques into my lifestyle has given me hope that I might be able to avoid future bowel adhesions and surgery. My symptoms have improved significantly, and I am convinced that the self-care massage and castor oil packs and dietary changes have given me a new lease on life. My husband and I are so thankful for this knowledge.

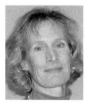

Jennifer O'Hagan RH (www.woodlandnaturals.com) Jennifer is a registered herbalist with the American Herbalists Guild and a certified practitioner and instructor of the Arvigo Techniques of Maya Abdominal Therapy® and Maya Spiritual Healing. She is a Loomis digestive health specialist, massage therapist, and Reiki master. She is the founder and president of Woodland Naturals and cofounder of the Changewater Wellness Center in Changewater, New Jersey. A past board member of the American Herbalists Guild, Jennifer served on the Advisory Council of the Arvigo Institute in Belize, Central America. Jennifer's additional certifications and trainings include Swedish massage, deep tissue massage, oncology and mastectomy massage, healthy breast massage, sports massage, reflexology, aromatherapy, pre- and post-natal massage, craniosacral,

visceral manipulation, shiatsu, and gua sha. She offers classes and lectures locally and internationally. Jennifer practices in Hope,
New Jersey.

Chronic Constipation   A common condition, chronic constipation is characterized by difficult, infrequent, or perceived incomplete evacuation of bowel movements. Symptoms include having fewer than three bowel movements per week, straining, hard stools, incomplete evacuation, and inability to pass stool. The prevalence of chronic constipation ranges from 2 to 28 percent; it increases with age and is more common in women than men. Constipation is caused by stool's spending too much time in the colon; the colon absorbs too much water from the stool, making it hard and dry, which makes it more difficult for the muscles of the rectum to push the stool out of the body. There are many different causes of chronic constipation: structural lesions of the colon (e.g., colon cancer, colon stricture, or narrowing); adhesions (bands of tissue that can connect the loops of the intestines to each other, which may block food or stool from moving through the GI tract); medical conditions (diabetes, thyroid disorders, Parkinson's disease, or pregnancy); medications (pain medications [narcotics], blood pressure medications [calcium channel blockers], antiseizure medication, and antispasmodics); and lifestyle issues (too little fiber, too little water, not enough exercise). Treatment for constipation depends on the cause, severity, and duration of the constipation and may include changes in eating, diet, and nutrition, exercise, and lifestyle, and medication. People who do not respond to these first-line treatments may be subject to additional tests, biofeedback, and surgery.

A Special Needs Child Finds Help with Digestion and Elimination

*To touch the surface is
to stir the depths.*

—DEANE JUHAN

Cristina (AS TOLD BY HER MOM) My 8-year-old daughter, Cristina, has cerebral palsy, sensory reactive disorder, and additional brain injury. She is able to walk with braces and support but is limited in her ability to communicate, showing dissatisfaction by pinching or pulling hair. She lets us know things are going well by looking deeply into our eyes while we're doing whatever we're doing. She has been making enormous strides in her treatments while working with professionals and specialists who are addressing her various needs.

I am very concerned about her digestion and elimination as she is often very constipated and goes several days without a bowel movement, causing her great discomfort and pain. It is very difficult to help this with diet changes as she will only eat certain foods. It is also a challenge to keep her hydrated unless she has cold drinks. I met Beth Townsend one day and she told me about Arvigo Therapy and the benefits it would have for my daughter. Also, Beth would teach me self-care massage in order for me to continue to help Cristina at home.

PRACTITIONER PERSPECTIVE   I adapted the Arvigo Therapy protocol using a light touch for Cristina's first session, knowing I had to be creative with my methods when working with children with special needs. In general, children are unable to remain still for extended periods of time. Developing trust with Cristina required me to work slowly and patiently.

Cristina was quiet and receptive while I performed the upper abdominal techniques and instructed her mom in the self-care massage. Craniosacral and Reiki therapy were used to help Cristina relax prior to the lower abdominal work which she readily received. During our session, there were times when she would look into my eyes, letting me know things were going well and something was working. This occurred several times during her treatment.

Cristina arrived for one of her sessions in pain associated with several days of constipation. She remained still for her treatment but about 75 percent of the way through she started to move. Her mom removed her so that she could thoroughly evacuate her bowel. This was significant and showed how things were "moving" for Cristina as a direct result of Arvigo Therapy.

Cristina's Mom's Experience   I was impressed with

Beth's sensitivity and patience while working with Cristina and when instructing me on how to do the self-care massage for her. I made sure that Cristina received the self care at home daily, and when elimination was becoming difficult, I would apply it more than once daily to prevent constipation. At Beth's recommendation, I was also able to help Cristina stay better hydrated by giving her more fluids but at room temperature which she tolerated well. As long as I continue to follow through with Cristina's self-care massage and fluid intake she no longer experiences pain or constipation. It has been many months now since our first session with Beth, and Arvigo Therapy has provided much comfort in Cristina's life and ours.

Beth Ann Townsend's professional biography appears on page 86.

Promoting Homeostasis Alleviates Lifelong Severe Chronic Constipation

I accept small gains, small victories, turning away from the idea that there is some quick fix that will make me feel heroic and invulnerable.

—JULIA CAMERON

Callie   I was born with a unique physical constitution with complications for which there was limited treatment. My childhood physicians and specialists were very invested in my well-being, but they were out of options for me. After many medical consultations, limited solutions were offered including more surgery that I was reluctant to have and a prescribed medication to relieve constipation, which rarely worked for me and more often aggravated the problem. After more than 20 years I made it a point to be my own best advocate and read whatever current applicable research I could find.

After viewing a Dr. Oz segment featuring stomach massage, I set out to find a similar treatment that could possibly treat my chronic severe constipation. My additional symptoms included constant low-grade nausea and physical discomfort, bloating, contracted menstrual cycle, and weak immunity. I had to closely monitor my food intake to ascertain what to eat and when to eat, with a limited diet of foods that would not worsen symptoms. Most mornings I felt ready to vomit until pressure in the bowels was decreased. Increasing fiber was not a solution for me: It made my symptoms worse! I happened upon the Arvigo Therapy website and made an appointment with a certified Arvigo practitioner. I had such a good feeling about the first encounter with Penny Ordway and Arvigo Therapy that I scheduled multiple future sessions.

PRACTITIONER PERSPECTIVE   Callie's medical history was daunting, extensive, and complex as she was born with cloacal anomaly. She presented with directional reversal of colon, extra slight loop in transverse colon, two uteri, and no coccyx. There was also scarring from multiple surgeries as an infant for kidney reflux and more surgeries throughout childhood. These additional procedures were to narrow part of the descending/sigmoid colon; to reconstruct the bladder and vaginal canal; to remove the appendix; and to implant mesh to support low back soft tissue structure.

Her endocrine system revealed abnormal thyroid, blood sugar, and estrogen levels, and her menstrual cycle was 21 to 23 days with fairly regular, near daily spotting. Ovulation and menstruation made the constipation and bloating worse. I ascertained the uteri to be a little low and difficult to distinguish at first. Her immune system was compromised: She tended to get sick easily and frequently. Eating too much fiber increased constipation. She presented with slight hernias around abdominal scars, aggravated by cinched clothing, tight waistbands, and by excessive constipation. Callie also suffered a head injury in the previous year, from which she had partially recovered.

Callie was committed to having a more normal life and was proactive in researching her best options. Included are some of her changes: a polyprobiotic regimen, keeping hydrated, eating organically, restricting her intake of foods and food combinations that were problematic. No matter how challenging, I knew working with Callie would be a genuine and positive partnership as she was very invested in her own health.

Arvigo Therapy sessions were initially scheduled for three to five times a week to restore tone and movement in the intestine and colon while enabling evacuation, reducing scar tissue, opening space in the abdomen to improve lymph gland functioning, and aligning reproductive organs. Manual lymphatic drainage was added to Arvigo Therapy sessions to further address the colon's functioning and reduce bloating.

At each session we were successful at reducing Callie's nausea and stimulating the bowel. Eventually, we added time for general effleurage and myofascial techniques for legs, arms, and upper back and some lymph drainage for the neck and head. Not only did this change her appearance to a more contoured face, it helped reduce her head-injury "fog." There were sessions where so much fluid moved out of the tissues and organs that I would stop three to twelve times for Callie to void her bladder! Upon return for her next session, Callie would report (happily) that the high volume fluid outflow had gone on for hours after the previous session.

Over the course of our time together, Callie and I achieved something phenomenal: bowels started to empty and be relatively regular; fluid retention decreased dramatically; and she lost significant weight and dropped several dress sizes. She ceased spotting almost entirely unless there were extraordinary circumstances like prolonged stress, sleep deprivation, episodes of constipation, air travel, or other interruptions in life's rhythm and routine. Her menstrual cycle adjusted to 25 to 28 days. Except for sporadic incidents, the general physical discomfort lessened or disappeared. Callie reported having more energy and clarity, and feeling happier overall. All these changes came about in a variety of ways: fits and starts, sometimes gradually and incrementally, or building one on the other and surprising us pleasantly at every turn.

Callie's Experience

My life has changed. I do not have the constant physical discomfort of feeling stuffed inside. Episodes with pain from herniated areas are gone. The thought that it's likely I have never had full bowel movements in the past is a revelation. I feel happier, and I don't know exactly how or why it happened, but my general hormone balance seems much improved. My waist is six inches smaller! Penny and I have been working on this for about sixteen months, and in that time, I have lost forty pounds. When

I see old pictures of myself, I see the wider torso and the water weight in my face and limbs. I don't even think about spotting as a concern so much anymore. Penny said our goal was to support and promote homeostasis. Her hope was that we could tone the colon and rebuild strength and peristaltic action while reducing the contents of my bowel to more normal volume. It was a simple approach that had the piggyback effect of all these great results. I still need the Arvigo Therapy; I still need to focus on my career and push through some tough times. But when I think back to how much harder my body had to work to maintain any kind of health, I have to say my experience with this genuinely powerful therapy and this dedicated practitioner is a real success story. More good things to come!

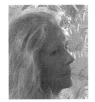 **Penny Ordway** (www.eviama.com) Penny Ordway has practiced healing arts for more than 30 years, beginning with MariEl, moving on to Reiki, organic skincare, manual lymph drainage, and a host of body therapies. The first time Rosita Arvigo introduced Maya abdominal work at a Green Nations gathering, Penny was there. She felt this straightforward but radical technique was a missing link for her healing work. She became certified in the Arvigo Techniques and Maya spiritual healing. Her holistic practice is tucked away in her sustainably designed green spa, graced with an open-air garden courtyard in the middle of urban Philadelphia.

A Comforting Regimen for Infant Acid Reflux

*A mother understands
what a child does not say.*

—JEWISH PROVERB

Jessica (AS TOLD BY HER MOM) My daughter Jessica is my third child, born full term via c-section due to her presenting butt first with the cord wrapped around her neck twice. She was very healthy, weighing in at 8 pounds, 4 ounces. Every time I breastfed her, she became gassy, spit up, or vomited. She was nursing every 2 hours, and about 95 percent of the time her stool was yellow and seedy. Our doctor recommended that I first supplement with different types of formula, but Jessica did not tolerate them any better. Next he prescribed several medications for her, planning to reassess her status at her 4 month checkup. Not being happy with this approach, I started looking into alternative therapies and found Christine Lee.

PRACTITIONER PERSPECTIVE Mom brought Jessica in to see me when she was 8 weeks old. She appeared quite healthy, with a robust cry, and I found her quite engaging! Her mom reviewed her symptoms with me as well as the medical doctor's treatment plan to try and wean Jessica off the medications once she reaches 4 months. Just this past week Jessica has started to sleep a 7-hour stretch.

In my experience I felt Arvigo Therapy would be appropriate for Jessica as her diaphragm may have become tucked up and stuck since the cord was around her neck during birth. Not having been born vaginally she did not receive the introduction of digestive bacteria into her gut. Jessica was and continues to be breastfed, so she was getting some good gut bacteria as colostrum is another source. I reviewed with mom the Arvigo Therapy modified for infants and using gentle strokes. I began to talk softly while working with Jessica and soon she was beginning to relate to her hands and feet; something Mom remarked that she hadn't seen her do with anyone outside the family so calmly before now. Mom was taught how to perform the self-care massage on Jessica's belly as well as some select strokes along the spine. We planned to stay in touch about Jessica's progress and having some follow-up sessions.

Jessica's Experience (IN HER "OWN" WORDS) It's been 3
weeks since Mommy took me to that nice lady Christine. I am amazed at how much better I am doing. I love it when Mommy rubs my belly and back and I am hoping I can stop taking that yucky tasting stuff the doctor told her to give me. We will find out if that's possible a month from now at my next checkup. I'm not spitting up as much, and I really like it when Daddy rubs my belly and back, too.

Mommy is amazed at how the belly massage is helping me. I'm amazed, too! Another 2 weeks have passed, and I can feel my legs relaxing more when she rubs my belly. I am spitting up less. Mommy does my massage first thing in the morning, and this helps me relax all over before I eat. I am still taking those yucky-tasting medicines, but the massage is helping and Mommy hopes I won't have to take the medicines for much longer. I am starting to be a much happier little camper!

Mommy is taking me to the doctor. I'm 4 months today, and I've been spitting up a bit more now and then. Why do parents freak out when we have these little setbacks? The doctor is changing my medicines, and I will be having something called an "endoscopy"— whatever that is. Mommy keeps doing my massage every day, and I just know that is helping me not to spit up as much.

Hooray! I'm 6 months old today, and I am no longer taking that yucky tasting medicine stuff. The doctor told Mommy that the test I had came back "negative." I'm loving life, Mommy's breast milk, and some very yummy stuff called baby food, oh, and of course, my time with Mommy and Daddy for my belly massage. "High 5" to Christine for teaching Mommy how to help me!

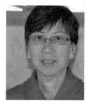 **Christine Lee** RNCS, Lic Ac, MSN, MAOM (www.acuchrisrn.com) Christine bridges the gap between Eastern and Western medicine by incorporating traditional healing modalities in providing holistic health care. Her family practice includes acupuncture, Reiki, cranio-sacral therapy, Arvigo Techniques of Maya Abdominal Therapy®, and herbal medicine. As a certified Arvigo therapy practitioner, Christine has discovered a deeper and greater faith in the body's ability to support healing physically, emotionally, and spiritually. Whether it's teaching Self Care classes, leading women's groups, or developing a deep breathing meditative practice, Christine shares her passion for self awareness and self care.

Infant Acid Reflux   Also called gastroesophageal reflux (GER), acid reflux is one of the most common causes of infant feeding problems. Around 25 percent of all babies experience some degree of it. Acid reflux can cause a range of conditions, from the mild (frequent, painless spitting up) to the severe (colic, abdominal pain, and frequent night waking), and is one of the most common causes of so-called colic. For cases of infant acid reflux, doctors often prescribe medicines to lessen the production of stomach acids.

Embracing Loss
Benefits Gastroparesis

Forgive everyone everything,
no matter what they've done,
including yourself.

—DR. ROSITA ARVIGO

Amanda Due to the sudden loss of one of my three children and unresolved trauma, I was suffering from gastroparesis which causes severe stomach pain along with other physical symptoms. I had lost significant weight and was unable to eat much or eliminate effectively. I was seeking help from allopathic medicine, homeopathy, a nutritionist, a naturopath, and a spiritual director before finding Christine Lee. During one of our first sessions, Christine taught me self-care abdominal massage. At that point I was uncomfortable with my own body, and experiencing a mind-body disconnect. I was very tentative about touching my own body, afraid of finding problems that I didn't want to face.

PRACTITIONER PERSPECTIVE   Amanda initially came to see me four years ago with a primary complaint of acid reflux, feeling like a burning at the back of her throat and tongue. She was 60 at the time, married with two children, and had a history of irritable bowel syndrome, with gas, bloating, and yellow stools when her digestion is poor. She had been restricting gluten, sugar, corn, carrots, bananas, teas, caffeine, and carbonated beverages from her diet as she knew that ingesting any of these foods would make her symptoms worse.

She also reported many other general symptoms associated with her digestive condition such as spontaneous sweating, lightheadedness, and dizziness when standing quickly. She had no appetite, was losing weight, found sleeping difficult, and had very low energy. Reproductive issues included a history of heavy menstrual periods with clotting, ovarian cyst, and the removal of a breast lump followed by radiation treatment. She does her best to keep active with resistance training, swimming, walking, and biking. She has arthritis of the neck and spine and takes numerous medications and supplements for her multiple conditions.

Her 19-year-old daughter died three years ago as a result of digestive issues similar to those Amanda was experiencing. Her daughter's condition developed over a short period of time, but she had always had "digestive issues."

When I first met Amanda, my initial impression was that she was compromised physically, emotionally, and spiritually. She appeared frozen and stagnated, and her digestive and elimination systems were responding to her stress. It seemed she was grieving the loss of her daughter but was unable to move forward after this devastating loss since her symptoms matched her daughter's. At one point she had developed an episode of fecal impaction requiring several emergency room visits to resolve.

Amanda's initial treatment plan included acupuncture and Arvigo Therapy sessions on a regular basis, allowing her ample time to integrate the session. She was taught self-care massage, use of castor oil packs to her abdomen, meditation, and spiritual bathing.

Over the four years we worked together, Amanda was also seeing her health care provider, gastroenterologist, spiritual director, couples counselor, nutritionist, EMDR therapist, and acupuncturist. Her progress was slow and steady. Over time, there was improvement with a combination of the services from practitioners and diligent self-care massage. Amanda is now able to eat and is gaining weight. It is important for her to be able to stay present in her body, obtain quality sleep, stay calm, and to eat regular meals as her symptoms are notably reduced. She is beginning to feel joy and is more engaged with her husband and sons.

Amanda's Experience
I have been experiencing Arvigo Therapy for four years now, and my symptoms and awareness have evolved. My sessions with Christine and my self-care massage have helped me to realize the gift of my womb and surrounding abdominal area instead of wanting to rip it out because the pain was so intense. I realize this is a part of my body that is wounded. My womb carried three children and held them with such care. Now it is empty and unnecessary. My abdomen is the first to react to the loss. Now I massage it with great care and gratitude and repeat the mantra of Ho'oponopono: "I'm sorry, forgive me, thank you, I love you." My body has served me well. As I do my self-care massage, I imagine a healthy, healing womb and abdomen. I am now able to feel areas of spasms where there is hurt and I massage especially gently there, trying to coax it away, to let go. I no longer feel the fear that I knew earlier and am more comfortable with my body, more attached now.

Christine Lee's professional biography appears on page 156.

Gastroparesis   A disease of the muscles of the stomach or the vagus nerve that controls the muscles, gastroparesis causes the muscles to stop working, resulting in inadequate grinding of food by the stomach, and poor emptying of food from the stomach into the intestine. It mostly affects women and can significantly impair their quality of life. If an underlying cause for the gastroparesis is identified, for example pancreatitis, the condition will subside when the underlying problem resolves. If there is no reversible cause, gastroparesis rarely resolves and may worsen with time. Despite extensive investigations, the majority of patients will suffer from gastroparesis without identifiable cause. Gastroparesis is best diagnosed by a nuclear medicine test called a gastric emptying study. The primary symptoms of gastroparesis are nausea and vomiting and, in severe cases, weight loss due to a reduced intake of food. Mild gastroparesis cases usually can be successfully managed with nutritional support (changing eating habits, size and frequency of meals, types of foods), drugs for treating nausea and vomiting, and drugs that stimulate the muscles to contract. Severe gastroparesis can require repeated hospitalizations to correct dehydration and malnutrition and to control symptoms. Surgery occasionally is used, the goal being to create a larger opening between the stomach and the intestine in order to aid the process of emptying the stomach's contents. Alternatively, the entire stomach may be removed. These procedures are considered only when all other measures have failed because surgical risks are high.

Disrupting the Formation Cycle of Post-Surgical Adhesions

> *It ain't over 'til it's over.*
>
> —YOGI BERRA

Tom   I am 44 years old and unfortunately no stranger to the operating table. It all started with three transurethral surgeries on my prostate (2002, 2007, 2009) and a surgery to remove a small bowel obstruction in 2010. After the bowel obstruction surgery I underwent three more surgeries within a 16-month span (July 2011, May 2012, October 2012) to remove abdominal adhesions that formed as a result of the bowel surgery. Also throw in another surgery in 2011 to remove a kidney stone stuck just below my bladder.

My frequent and severe abdominal and pelvic pain came on after the three major surgeries to remove adhesions. Each surgery required at least two months to recover. I knew I had to break the cycle somehow, and went to many different hospitals seeking help. I had a long list of doctors, from some of the nation's best hospitals, all telling me, essentially, to give up. I was told there was nothing I could do to improve my situation, and that any such effort was a waste of time.

PRACTITIONER PERSPECTIVE   When I first met Tom, he was fearful and anxious at the potential for more bowel obstructions and adhesions as a result of past surgeries; he also had other symptoms such as frequent urination, weak stream, painful ejaculation, and chronic pelvic floor pain. He was born with an

161

intestinal birth defect (Meckel's diverticulum), which was diagnosed with the onset of the abdominal pain prior to his bowel obstruction surgery. He rates his daily pain at 3 to 8 on a scale of 10, with 10 being the worst. The pain is often in the lower abdomen, from the center stretching over a couple of inches to his right side; it becomes worse with prolonged sitting. He has been under the care of a primary physician and a urologist, and will have a consultation at Cleveland Clinic. Other treatments include chiropractic care, myofascial therapy (internal and external), stretching, lidocaine cream, hot packs, and cold packs, all of which offer temporary relief. He describes himself as spiritual, somewhere between Taoism and Buddhism.

When I examined Tom, I noticed a long abdominal scar extending from 1 inch above the navel to just above the pubic bone; the lower 4 to 5 inches of the scar were slightly pink in comparison to rest of the scar. His hips were tight; there was a leg length discrepancy; and he had very tight quadratus lumborum muscles bilateral.

I felt the abdominal and chronic pelvic floor pain were related and wanted to explore using Arvigo Therapy to work with his respiratory diaphragm to relax and release his pelvic diaphragm. Our initial plan included Arvigo Therapy sessions weekly for one month, then every other week for 2 months, and monthly for a few months longer. Tom also received acupuncture and herbal treatments from me for the first month. We discussed aspects of self care and how to do it at home, including daily self-care massage, applying castor oil packs daily for 2 months (decreasing this over time), diaphragmatic breathing, and squatting exercises.

In addition, I consulted with Karl Monahan, an Arvigo Practitioner in the UK who specializes in working with men. Karl suggested that Tom consider supplementing with vitamin C to reduce inflammation and magnesium as a muscle relaxant in addition to the probiotics he was taking.

Within a few months after starting Arvigo Therapy, Tom's abdominal pain was down to 3 or 4 on the 10-point scale, and it happened no more than two days a week. When I examined him, his abdominal scar felt softer and appeared less pink. His pelvic bones were well aligned, and his musculature was more even and soft.

Tom's Experience

Don't give up! There are answers out there if you look for them. Arvigo Therapy has been extremely beneficial for my situation. Christine has provided excellent guidance on how to care for myself at home, as well as nutrition suggestions and advice on supplements. I learned that there is no one "silver bullet" for treating my condition, and Christine has done a wonderful job of developing a highly effective strategy for me that integrates a variety of steps. I am feeling healthier and stronger than I have in years, and it is a direct result of Christine's help.

Christine Lee's professional biography appears on page 156.

Appendix

Humble Beginnings around the Kitchen Table

EVERY ORGANIZATION has it humble beginnings, and ours is no different. From the traditional healers of Belize, Dr. Rosita Arvigo, DN, was able to integrate the science with the traditional healing practices she learned. She treated many clients in her clinic in San Ignacio, and at Ix Chel Farm (now part of Chaa Creek Lodge in Belize). It was through her experiences that Arvigo Therapy has grown in 15 years to what it is today, a global community of dedicated practitioners!

Colletta Aberdale was Dr. Arvigo's first program organizer. In the winter of 1995, she met Rosita at a talk and book signing of *Sastun* at Smith College, Northampton, Massachusetts. Immediately, she felt a strong connection to the story and traveled to Ix Chel Farm that spring with an herbal group. At this time Colletta spoke with Rosita about the possibility of applying to volunteer at the farm for the fall of 1995. Her application was submitted, and, much to her amazement, she was accepted when an unexpected opening for this coveted position became available. As a clinical social worker at a teaching medical center in Western Massachusetts, she obtained a leave of absence and headed to Belize for a three- to six-month commitment.

Colletta spent the time from September 1995 to April 1996 as a volunteer, assisting in a wide range of duties such as farm chores, providing guided tours of the medicine trail to tourists, assisting with groups who visited Ix Chel Farm including Rosita's educational herbal groups, spiritual healing, etc. During this time she had the opportunity to meet with Don Elijio Panti while driving Rosita to his home/clinic. Colletta and Rosita formed a deep friendship, and discussions began around the kitchen table about developing "Maya Uterine massage," which this technique was known as at that time.

In 1996 Rosita began teaching Self Care workshops at many herbal conferences in the U.S. In a short time the program was formed, branching into three phases: Self Care, Professional training, and Certification training. Some traveled to Belize to attend the trainings, which were also taught in many states. Colletta was the coordinator for these trainings and was responsible for marketing and selling Rainforest Remedies when the product was introduced in the U.S. Within a few years Colletta felt the program would benefit from a full-time practitioner to assume these responsibilities, and Diane MacDonald became program administrator in 2002. And the program did indeed grow over many years!

Colletta currently maintains her private psychotherapy practice in Western Massachusetts and remains in touch with many of the wonderful women she met through the years. As she states: "The experience was very rewarding and life changing for me."

From 2002 to present, the Arvigo Institute, LLC, continues to develop by leaps and bounds from the early days of a small office in Diane and Steve MacDonald's spare room to a real office outside of their home in rural Antrim, New Hampshire. The Arvigo Institute, LLC, is a licensed post-secondary school in New Hampshire and a national provider of continuing education for midwives, massage therapists, and acupuncturists. To date, more than 2,500 Arvigo practitioners have been trained, representing more than 20 countries around the globe. Since Rosita retired from teaching Self Care and professional classes, the demand for quality education has risen. We now have 50 certified teachers in 8 countries and more to come.

Humble beginnings, to be sure, but with the intent to ensure future generations continue to have access hundreds of years from now to this remarkable traditional therapy that is hundreds of years old.

About Ix Chel:
Maya Goddess of Medicine,
Weaving, and Childbirth

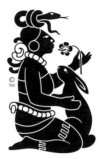

In 1986, on one of our very first forays into the jungle searching for medicinal plants, Don Elijio said that "walking in the mountains with a woman was very good luck." We trudged farther up the mountainside toward the rising sun. "Ix Chel shows her medicine more readily when a healer walks with a woman." Out of breath trundling along behind him, I asked, "Who is Ix Chel?" Patiently, as if speaking to a child, he answered, "She is the Goddess of healing. Women pray to her for fertility, and she brings dream visions to healers and weavers. She is my very best friend."

—Rosita Arvigo, DN

In Maya, *Ix* means goddess or the feminine sacred; *Chel* means rainbow or light. Ix Chel was also known as Lady Rainbow, Goddess of the Rainbow, or Lady of the Sacred Light. In glyphs she wears a snake. The snake has been a symbol of medicine and healing for many ancient cultures around the world, including the Maya, Aztec, Greek, Roman, Egyptian, Druid, East Indian, and African, and continues to be a symbol in medical professional fields such as the American Medical Association's symbol of the caduceus, a winged staff with two snakes.

Taking Care of Yourself

*Big, sweeping life changes
really boil down to small
everyday decisions.*

—ALI VINCENT

HOW DO WE NOURISH ourselves on a physical, emotional, and spiritual level each and every day? What are some activities that you can add to your daily routine that will enhance your health and wellness while also nourishing and nurturing your soul? Perhaps you take time each day to enjoy a walk outside, journal your thoughts, take a yoga class, paint, or participate in another enjoyable activity. Many people, however, fret that there is not enough time to do such activities as they scramble hectically from one appointment to another, juggling job, parenting, and childcare or eldercare commitments.

The World Health Organization defines self care as "activities individuals, families, and communities undertake with the intention of enhancing health, preventing disease, limiting illness, and restoring health. These activities are derived from knowledge and skills from the pool of both professional and lay experience. They are undertaken by lay people on their own behalf, either separately or in participative collaboration with professionals." Other experts define self care in terms of individual behavior when a person functions on his or her own behalf in health promotion and prevention or in disease detection and treatment. In this definition, self care behaviors occur without professional assistance, but individuals are informed by technical knowledge and skills derived from both professional and lay experience. Still others define self care as involving activities to enhance health, prevent disease, evaluate symptoms, and restore health—either with or without participation by professionals. Whatever definition of self care resonates with you, all three definitions above have a similar theme: Self care consists of activities one does to enhance and restore heath and prevent disease.

One component is evident in all of the case studies in this book. The Arvigo practitioners supported their clients' health and wellness issues in ways that went beyond the clients' receiving professional sessions. Each practitioner taught the client self-care massage and encouraged the client to bring her/his healing hands to the body. Each client was committed to self care. Self-care massage techniques are the cornerstone of ATMAT, integral to professional practitioner sessions and bringing clients closer and deeper into their own healing process.

In the following pages you will read about an Arvigo practitioner's personal experience with self care massage. You will find general information and instructions on self care massage; castor oil pack and vaginal steam bath application; how to make and use a faja; and how to offer yourself a spiritual herbal bath. These are simple and inexpensive to apply and readily accessible, yet they are powerful tools that can nurture and nourish the core of your being. Being consistent with your self care is important because it's the small things you do every day on a regular basis that will make the most difference for you.

Please note that the information in this section does not replace consulting with your health care provider or an Arvigo practitioner. To find a qualified practitioner near you, visit www.arvigotherapy.com.

BELLY LOVE

I've probably done close to 7,000 abdominal massages over the years and I find that every single belly is absolutely beautiful and unique, and has a story to tell.

When I massage wrinkled, sun-spotted hands, I think about how many tears those hands have wiped dry, flowers they have planted, hands they have tenderly held, meals they have prepared. When I massage arms, I think of how they have embraced and comforted those in need. And with bellies, I think about the sweet life that grew inside or the sadness and heartache held within.

Just for a moment, think about the history your body has experienced. What is the first thing that comes to mind? I remember years ago, during my training as an Arvigo practitioner, Dr. Rosita Arvigo was working on my "cement post." The cement post is the area between your xiphoid process and navel, also known as the solar plexus. It's the area where you get that sinking feeling when something shocking or hurtful happens. When emotions aren't processed, this area can feel hard like a cement post. As Rosita massaged this area on me, a memory came up from my childhood. An image of two boys in a stairwell, and they were laughing at me and calling me stupid. I felt ashamed and belittled. I don't ever recall having this memory before. It just popped up in the moment Rosita was massaging my belly. Rosita asked if I was okay. I wasn't crying or anything, but in her loving way she nodded her head, knowing something old and painful was moving out. When emotions come up during a session, I tell my clients what Rosita told me, "Just observe the energy/feeling/emotion, not trying to figure it out, just watch and feel. Observe it as you would a train going by. You can see how fast it's going and what color it is, but you don't have to get on the train and no one has to get off. Just allow it to go by."

The interesting thing is, feeling stupid was a recurring feeling I had experienced most of my life. I felt insecure about my intelligence even though I did well in school. I know I have been ignorant about many things in life, and I'm hyper aware when people have recognized my naiveté. I've registered and stored every eye roll or condescending laugh as a confirmation that I'm not good enough, smart enough, or lovable. I think the memory that came up that day was an accumulation of 35-plus years of all of those moments. This belief that I was stupid affected how I carried my body, the life choices I made, and how I acted in social situations.

Abdominal self-care massage helped me process and move out those old emotional charges. Restorative Exercise™ helped me as well. I feel freer in my body and more confident now.

Now think about how amazing your body is, physiologically speaking. Really think about how hard your body is working for you. All the biochemical reactions, biofeedback systems, cellular regeneration, waste elimination, pH balancing, attacking foreign invaders, and delivering oxygen and nutrients to every single cell in the body. The liver alone has more than 500 known biological functions! (It's not just for processing alcohol.) The body is beautifully designed and is performing an exquisite symphony of biochemical reactions to maintain balance within. Billions of communications and reactions every second as you sit on the couch watching back-to-back episodes of *Untold Stories of the E.R.* I love that show! Instead of sitting on the couch, I lie on the floor in a psoas release or spinal twist while watching it because I love my internal organs.

Oftentimes a physical problem is a healthy response to an unhealthy situation. The most rewarding part of my job is when I see someone accept and appreciate the wisdom of their physical body. Abdominal self-care massage allows you to connect to your body's wisdom. Many people who come in for treatments are angry at their bodies for causing them pain, fertility challenges, or for basically "not working correctly." Rude, insensitive people aren't the only ones who can impact you physically and emotionally with harsh words. Take a look at the messages you're sending to your own body throughout the day. Take time to smile down gratitude to your liver, uterus, or heart. Feel that smiling energy warm your entire body and then just listen as you would listen to a good friend.

—Barbara Loomis, LMT, RES
February 11, 2014

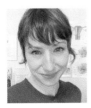 **Barbara Loomis** LMT, RES (www.nurturance.net) Barbara Loomis is a Restorative Exercise™ specialist and holds dual certifications in abdominal therapy. She is a certified practitioner and educator of the Arvigo Techniques of Maya Abdominal Therapy® as well as a certified Chi Nei Tsang (Chinese abdominal therapy) practitioner and Visceral Manipulation™ therapist. Her practice, Nurturance, is located in Portland, Oregon.

SELF-CARE MASSAGE

ALTHOUGH IT'S BEST to work with a trained Arvigo practitioner, anyone can learn the self-care massage technique described here. You may experience some temporary changes in menstruation, including a heavier blood flow or an increase in the number of days of flow. This is a sign that your uterus is cleansing. If you become pregnant, stop self-care massage and seek the advice of a trained Arvigo practitioner for prenatal massage techniques.

To locate Arvigo workshops and/or practitioner in your area, go to http:// arvigotherapy.com

Cautions and Contraindications: While this technique is safe when applied appropriately, there are times when direct massage over the uterus is contraindicated. Do not perform direct massage on your uterus if you are pregnant; have had abdominal surgery within the last six months; are under medical treatment for cancer or pelvic infection; or wear an intrauterine device (IUD) for birth control. Do not continue with self-care massage if you should experience pain or emotional upheavals during the treatment; are taking any painkillers that might mask pain during treatment; or experience a sudden onset of pain. Refer to your health care provider or Arvigo practitioner for appropriate evaluation.

Directions

- Wear loose, comfortable clothes. Empty your bladder. Lie on your back, with support under your knees.
- Relax and breathe deeply for several minutes.
- Bring both hands together onto the pubic bone. Tuck one thumb under the other, with the other eight fingers close together. Fingers should be slightly bent and relaxed so that your hands resemble a hoe.
- Slide your hands off the pubic bone toward your navel, and sink your fingers as deep into the soft flesh as is comfortable.
- On your next exhalation, firmly stroke in an upward motion halfway to your navel. Remember to breathe slowly and exhale with each massage

stroke. Repeat this upward movement of your hands, from pubic bone toward navel, for about two minutes.

- If you experience discomfort, reduce the pressure but continue to massage upward and within your comfort zone. If you experience any tenderness after the massage, give yourself a few days' rest before resuming self massage using a lighter touch.

HEALING WITH CASTOR OIL PACKS

CASTOR OIL is derived from the bean of the *Ricinus communis* plant, also called *Palma Christi* (palm of Christ). The Palma Christi has been used therapeutically for centuries in folk medicine of ancient India, China, Persia, Africa, Greece, Rome, and the Americas. It has large, beautiful palmate leaves, hence the name, Palma Christi.

Edgar Cayce, a medical intuitive known as the "sleeping prophet," introduced castor oil packs for the treatment of many conditions.

Some of the numerous uses of castor oil include the treatment of breast cysts, fibroids, ovarian cysts, congestion of abdominal organs, skin conditions, small benign cysts, and adhesions from surgery. Wherever there is congestion, scar tissue, decreased blood flow, and need for healing, castor oil can be an effective treatment option.

How does castor oil work?

Research has shown castor oil has a unique chemical profile rich in ricinoleic acid which is found only in the castor bean from which the oil is extracted. Double-blind studies conducted by the Association for Research and Enlightenment, Inc., demonstrated an increase in lymphocyte production and the level of activity of T-cell lymphocytes in the group that used castor oil packs. T-cell lymphocytes originate from bone marrow and the thymus gland. They identify and kill invaders such as viruses, bacteria, and fungi.

In addition to strengthening the immune system, castor oil appears to have a balancing effect on the autonomic nervous system, increasing liver activity and improving digestion. Tumors, fibroids, and cysts can be shrunken and eliminated by reabsorption.

What is a castor oil pack?

The standard pack recommended by Edgar Cayce consists of several layers of white wool flannel (because it holds heat better), but cotton flannel is also used with excellent results. Castor oil is soaked on the material and applied to the area in need of healing.

How is a castor oil pack used?

Warm the castor oil to skin temperature in a nonmetallic pot. Soak the flannel in the oil to make it well saturated but not dripping. Place the pack over the area to be treated, and cover the pack with plastic food wrap. Place a heat source, a heating pack or hot water bottle, on top of the pack to maintain consistent warmth throughout the treatment. Secure this in place with a heavy towel.

While the pack is working, quietly meditate to connect the mind and body healing energies. This assists the spiritual essence of the plant to assist in your healing. Often people find the thoughts that occur in this meditative state are as important as the properties of the oil to their healing process. Write in your journal the thoughts, feelings, or images that may occur during this treatment.

Adjust the heat setting to your comfort. ***Do not fall asleep while using the heating pad.*** Continue treatment for one hour. An alternative to using the pack with a heat source: Secure pack with a towel wrapped around your body, secure with pins, and leave in place overnight.

How do I prevent staining from the oil?

To protect bedding or clothing from staining, plastic sheets from dry-cleaning bags, old plastic table cloths, old shower curtains, old heavy bath towels, and the like are typically effective. Baking soda may be used during laundering to remove some of the stains on fabric.

How are the packs maintained?

To reuse a pack for multiple treatments, just resaturate with oil. A pack can be stored in a plastic bag or glass jar for six months to a year as long as it does not become rancid or soiled. Packs should not be shared with other persons.

How often do I use the packs as a treatment?

A typical regimen for non-acute conditions is three times a week, every other night for three weeks with the fourth week off. Repeat this for two more cycles, take a week off, and then continue once a week or until symptoms subside.

For acute conditions, use for 30 minutes nightly for five nights, take two nights off, then repeat the cycle for two weeks or until the condition is resolved.

Are there any contraindications to usage?

Do not use the packs during times of heavy bleeding, gaseous stomach, intestinal conditions, or during pregnancy.

On rare occasion a rash may occur at the site. This is a normal occurrence of the body's way to eliminate toxins. Cleanse the area with a solution of one tablespoon baking soda to one cup of warm water.

HERBAL VAGINAL STEAM

VAGINAL STEAM BATHS, or *bajos* (BAH-hoes), as they are known in Spanish, are used to assist in the cleansing of the uterus in conjunction with the Arvigo Therapy for the treatment of numerous female symptoms.

Plants: The most commonly used are marigold, oregano, basil, rosemary, motherwort, St. John's wort, chamomile, damiana, red clover, dandelion, yellow dock, squaw vine, horsetail, and Mexican wormseed *(epazote)*.

Directions:
- Collect plants using prayer and a clear intention of healing. If using fresh plant, use about 1 quart; if using dry, about a cup.
- In a large pot containing about a gallon of water, place the above plants. Crush the herbs into the water, thanking them for helping with your healing.

- Offer prayers nine times. These prayers can be to whatever Spirit offers you guidance (Goddess, Jesus, Christ, God, Mother Earth, Father in Heaven, etc.). Most important are the prayer, faith, and intention.
- Bring this to a soft boil for 5 minutes; steep for 10 minutes with the lid on.
- With the pot under a slatted chair, lawn chair, etc., sit on the chair without underwear.
- Wear socks to keep your feet warm, draping fully with a blanket around your waist to the floor. Be careful not to allow any draft underneath you. Be sure you are enclosed by the blankets from the waist down and in something warm from the waist up.
- Sitting quietly over your pot of herbal steam for 20 minutes, meditate, read, enjoy, and find pleasure in the herbal healing. The heat should feel warming and pleasant. If it is too warm, remove the pot for a few minutes.
- After the vaginal steam bath, wrap yourself in the blanket, allowing a time of rest and meditation for about 20 minutes or so. Be careful not to expose yourself to cool drafts or temperature changes.
- Depending upon the condition you are treating, vaginal steam baths are done prior to menses or just after. Expect changes in your vaginal discharge and menstruation. These are normal cleansing reactions.
- Inform your practitioner if you have any unusual discharge or response to this treatment.

HOW TO MAKE AND USE THE FAJA

THE FAJA (FAH-ha) is a cloth band worn by Central American women to support their uteri. The following are general directions to make and wear the faja either for yourself or for your clients:

- Plain cotton muslin cloth works best. Cut a strip about 12 inches wide and 3 to 4 yards long that is sufficient to wrap around the pelvis with enough left over to tie a knot or tuck in the ends. Adjust the length of the faja as needed to meet the needs of the body. A piece of an old cotton sheet or shawl works well too.

- Place the faja on a flat surface. Lie down on the cloth with your low back in the center of the cloth. You will have the two long sides on either side of your body. Wrap the cloth firmly around your abdomen, wrapping it around the pelvis firmly and securely. Give a twist in the back and bring the two ends around to the front to tie in a lateral or medial position that will best support the uterus. The faja is worn all day under the underwear.
- Check to ensure the faja is not too tight. If your legs tingle, feel numb, or turn bluish, loosen the knot to allow circulation to and from the extremities.
- Wearing a faja supports the uterus to allow the body time to repair uterine ligaments and increase circulation and nerve supply to the organs and surrounding tissues. This takes anywhere from 24 hours to 30 days.
- When wearing the faja, avoid wearing high-heeled shoes, running, high-impact exercise classes, lifting heavy objects, horseback riding, or other strenuous activity. Overstretching of the ligaments is counterproductive to healing.
- Be patient! The self-care massage and faja always help. Some clients choose to wear the faja for a day or two before their menses begin in order to alleviate that feeling of heaviness. Others just wear it because they like the way it makes them feel.

IMPORTANT: *Do not wear the faja at night or during menses!*

SPIRITUAL HERBAL BATHING

HERBAL BATHS have been used by Maya healers for centuries to refresh the body and purify the electromagnetic field surrounding each person. The combination of the power of water, prayer, intention, and healing properties of the plants provides deep cleansing and renewal at an energetic level. Collect your plants with prayer and intention in preparation for your bath.

Plants: Choose plants for your bath that will bring meaning and healing for you as each plant brings its own healing wisdom. Commonly used plants are lavender, oregano, basil, marigold, rose, yarrow, lemon balm, hibiscus, St. John's wort, echinacea, or any nontoxic plant that resonates with you.

Directions:

- Fresh herbs: Place 2 gallons of water and 1 quart of herbs in a large bucket. Crush the herbs with both hands into the water, offering your prayers and thanks to the water and plants that aid in your healing. Be specific so they are clear about your healing request and intention. Place in direct sunlight for a few hours if possible.
- Dried herbs: Use 2 cups of dried plants in 2 gallons of hot water, and steep until desired temperature for bathing. Crush the plants in the water with your hands while saying prayers appropriate for you.
- Use incense such as copal, sage, or other resin to aid in clearing and centering.
- Take a sip of the herbal water. Begin to meditate on your healing.
- Slowly scoop and splash the herbal bath water over yourself with a bowl or cup, reserving enough to do a foot soak. Place your feet in the herbal water for about 10 minutes while you pray and meditate.
- If bathing in the shower or tub, strain the water off into another container so that the bathroom drain doesn't get clogged up. If you can bathe outside, no need to worry about straining the bath water.

Rest, meditate, journal—be with yourself in this healing way!

RAINFOREST REMEDIES

No healer can work alone to cure people. Our tools are plants, prayers, and faith in God.

—DON ELIJIO PANTI

RAINFOREST REMEDIES is a cooperative company located in Belize, Central America. Formulations are drawn directly from the centuries-old Mayan healing traditions and gathered from soil rich in calcium and minerals from the rainforest of Belize. Rainforest Remedies represents Dr. Arvigo's work to preserve both the library of traditional healing and the rainforest for the benefit of ecology and mankind. The herbs in Rainforest Remedies formulations are harvested from uncultivated areas already scheduled for clearing and development. Dr Arvigo refers to this as "salvage botany; harvesting valuable medicinal plants that would otherwise be destroyed." As prescribed by ancient Mayan traditions, the herbs are always gathered by herb collectors in traditional ways and with traditional prayers.

The rainforest of the Yucatan peninsula is a unique herbal environment. Many of the herbs in the formulations were unknown to most of the world until quite recently. The books *Rainforest Remedies: 100 Healing Herbs of Belize* and *Sastun* are references for further learning about the plants. Herbal formulas are sent to the Arvigo Institute office in New Hampshire in small batches to ensure the highest quality possible. For more information visit www.arvigo-therapy.com and click on Rainforest Remedies for a complete list of products.

Practitioners of the Arvigo Techniques incorporate herbal support according to client needs and the practitioner's license and/or scope of practice as governed by where they work. As noted by some of the case studies in this book, use of herbal support, along with the self-care massage and other supportive modalities, provides relief of symptoms. Consult with your practitioner or health care provider prior to using the formulations.

As a distributor of Rainforest Remedies the Arvigo Institute, LLC, makes clear that the U.S. Food and Drug Administration has not evaluated these formulations nor the statements the Arvigo Therapy program makes about them. We make no claim that these formulations diagnose, treat, cure, or prevent disease as they have not undergone scientific studies. Our information is based on centuries of traditional use, practitioner experience, and studies of which we are aware.

Glossary

Acupuncture is a system of complementary medicine that involves penetration of the skin with needles to stimulate certain points on the body to treat various physical, mental, and emotional conditions. According to traditional Chinese medicine, stimulating these specific acupuncture points corrects imbalances in the flow of qi (life force) through channels known as meridians (paths through which qi flows).

Adhesions are fibrous bands that form between tissues and organs, often as a result of injury during surgery. They form as a natural part of the body's healing process after surgery in the same way that a scar forms. They can be thought of as internal scar tissue that connects tissues and other body structures not normally connected.

Allopathic medicine is mainstream, Western medicine.

Antalgic is a posture or gait adopted by an individual to minimize or avoid pain.

Anteflexed uterus is a uterus that is tilted forward in the abdominal cavity.

ASIS (anterior superior iliac spine) is a projection at the anterior end of the iliac crest.

Assisted reproductive technology (ART) comprises several types of medical treatment designed to result in pregnancy.

Bacterial vaginosis (BV) is the most common cause of vaginal infection for women of childbearing age, caused by imbalance of naturally occurring bacterial flora.

Bajos is an herbal and steam facial for the vagina.

Benign prostatic hyperplasia (BPH) is a common urological condition caused by the noncancerous enlargement of the prostate gland as men get older.

183

C-section (caesarean section) is a surgical procedure in which one or more incisions are made through a mother's abdomen and uterus to deliver one or more babies.

Cloacal anomalies refers to a collection of defects that occur during fetal development in a female's lower abdominal structures. There are many variations to these defects; the most common involve a merging of the rectum, genital tract (vagina), and urinary tract (urethra) into one exit out of the body.

Coccyx commonly refers to the tailbone and consists of three or more small bones fused together at the bottom of the spine.

Cognitive behavioral therapy (CBT) is a type of psychotherapeutic treatment that helps patients understand the thoughts and feelings that influence behaviors to improve coping. CBT is commonly used to treat a wide range of disorders including phobias, addiction, depression, and anxiety.

Colitis is swelling (inflammation) of the large intestine (colon).

CPPS See Prostatitis.

Craniosacral therapy is a form of bodywork therapy that uses light therapeutic touch to help regulate the flow of cerebrospinal fluid to promote healing.

Cerebral palsy is a condition marked by impaired muscle coordination (spastic paralysis) and/or other disabilities, typically caused by damage to the brain before or during birth.

D&C (dilation and curettage) refers to the dilation of the cervix and surgical removal of part of the lining of the uterus and/or contents of the uterus by scraping and scooping.

Dysmenorrhea is painful menstruation, typically involving abdominal cramps.

Dysplasia of the hip is a congenital or developmental deformation or misalignment of the hip joint.

EMDR (eye movement desensitization and reprocessing) is a psychotherapy treatment designed to alleviate the distress associated with traumatic memories.

Endometriosis is a condition resulting from the retrograde flow of endometrial cells out of the fallopian tubes into the lower pelvic cavity and abdomen. The endometrial cells start to adhere to the surrounding organs and bleed during menses, causing pain and adhesions.

Endoscopy is a nonsurgical procedure in which a flexible tube is inserted to examine and take pictures of a person's digestive tract.

Faja (FAH-ha) is a Central American belly wrap used to support abdominal and reproductive organs; it is usually made of cotton muslin.

Female Tonic is an herbal tincture traditionally used to support and cleanse the uterus. Don Elijio Panti's original formula is sold by Rainforest Remedies in Belize.

Fundus of the uterus is the top portion, opposite from the cervix. Fundal height, measured from the top of the pubic bone, is routinely measured in pregnancy.

Gastroparesis is a condition in which the stomach can't empty food properly.

Gluten is a substance present in some grains, especially wheat, that is responsible for the elastic texture of dough.

Gluten sensitivity/intolerance is a spectrum of disorders, including celiac disease and wheat allergy, in which gluten has an adverse effect on the body. Symptoms include bloating, abdominal discomfort or pain, diarrhea, muscular disturbances, and bone or joint pain.

H'men (one who knows) is the doctor-priest/priestess who has the ability to heal in both the physical and spiritual realms.

Hemodynamics refers to the dynamics of blood circulation.

Homeopathy is an alternative medical practice in which extremely dilute amounts of certain natural substances are used to treat various ailments.

Homeostasis is the property of a living organism to regulate its internal environment to maintain a stable condition by means of adjustments controlled by interrelated regulatory mechanisms.

Ho'oponopono is an ancient Hawaiian practice of reconciliation and forgiveness.

Hysterosalpingogram (HSG) is an x-ray of the uterus and Fallopian tubes to see if there are any blockages; usually performed in diagnosing infertility.

IBS (irritable bowel syndrome) is a widespread condition involving recurrent abdominal pain and diarrhea or constipation, often associated with stress, depression, anxiety, or previous intestinal infection.

Ischium is the curved bone forming the base of each half of the pelvis.

IVF (in vitro fertilization) involves combining eggs and sperm outside the body in a laboratory. Once an embryo forms, it is then placed in the uterus.

IUI (intrauterine insemination) is an infertility treatment that is often called artificial insemination. In this procedure, specially prepared sperm are inserted into the woman's uterus. Sometimes the woman is treated with medicines that stimulate ovulation before IUI.

IUD (intrauterine device) is a small, T-shaped device made of flexible plastic that is inserted into a woman's uterus to prevent pregnancy. The IUD is either wrapped in copper or contains hormones.

Kegel exercises are a set of special exercises that strengthen the pelvic floor.

Laparoscopy is a surgical procedure in which a fiber-optic instrument is inserted through the abdominal wall to view the organs in the abdomen or to permit a surgical procedure. It is the most common procedure used to diagnose and remove mild to moderate endometriosis.

Meckel's diverticulum is a slight bulge in the lower part of the small intestine; it is present at birth.

Naprapathy is the treatment of disease by manipulation of joints, muscles, and ligaments, based on the belief that many diseases are caused by displacement of connective tissues.

Naturopathy is a system of alternative medicine steeped in traditional healing methods, principles, and practices. Its practitioners focus on holistic, proactive prevention and comprehensive diagnosis and treatment without the use of pharmaceuticals.

Nerve Tonic is an herbal tincture formula traditionally used to support the nervous system; distributed in the U.S. by Rainforest Remedies.

PCOS (polycystic ovary syndrome) is the most common female endocrine disorder; it involves multiple organ systems and is believed to be fundamentally caused by insensitivity to the hormone insulin.

Pessary is a removable device that is placed into the vagina to support areas of pelvic organ prolapse.

Pitocin is a synthetic form of oxytocin used to induce labor. Oxytocin is the natural hormone released by the mother's pituitary gland that causes increased contraction of the uterus during labor and stimulates the ejection of milk into the ducts of the breasts.

PMS (premenstrual syndrome) refers to a wide range of symptoms that start the second half of the menstrual cycle and go away within one to two days after the period starts.

Procidentia is a medical term similar to prolapse, the falling down of an organ from its normal anatomical position.

Prolapse is a common condition that occurs when the structures designed to keep organs in place weaken or stretch, causing them to slip forward or down.

Prostatitis is inflammation of the prostate. Chronic prostatitis and chronic pelvic pain syndrome (CPPS) are the most common types of prostatitis.

PSA (prostate-specific antigen) is a protein produced exclusively by prostate cells. A simple blood test to measure a man's PSA level may help to detect early prostate cancer.

Pudendal nerve is a nerve in the pelvic region that carries sensory and motor fibers. It innervates the external genitalia of both sexes, as well as sphincters for the bladder and rectum.

Quadratus lumborum is a muscle in the lower back.

Rainforest Remedies are herbal remedies formulated in Belize by Dr. Rosita Arvigo based on traditional healing; distributed in the U.S.

Reiki is a healing technique based on the principle that the therapist can channel energy into the patient by means of touch, to activate the natural healing processes of the patient's body and restore physical and emotional well-being.

Relaxin is a hormone produced by the ovaries during pregnancy that causes pelvic and cervical expansion and relaxation.

Retroverted uterus means the uterus is tipped backward so that it aims toward the rectum instead of forward toward the belly.

Secondary infertility is defined as the inability to become pregnant, or to carry a pregnancy to term, following the birth of one or more biological children.

Spiritual bath combines the power of water, prayer, intention, and healing properties of plants for deep cleansing and renewal at an energetic level. Herbal spiritual baths have been used by Maya healers for centuries.

Stress incontinence is unintentional or uncontrollable leakage of urine when pressure within the abdomen increases suddenly, as in coughing, sneezing, or jumping.

Transvaginal ultrasound is a type of pelvic ultrasound involving insertion of a probe into the vagina to look at a woman's reproductive organs, including the uterus, ovaries, cervix, and vagina.

UTI (urinary tract infection), also known as acute cystitis, or bladder infection, is usually a bacterial infection that affects the urinary system.

Varicocele is an enlargement of the veins in the scrotum.

VBAC (vaginal birth after caesarean) is the practice of birthing a baby vaginally after a previous baby has been delivered through caesarean section. According to the American Pregnancy Association, 90 percent of women who have undergone caesarean births are candidates for VBAC.

Recommended Reading

*To know that we know what
we know, and to know that we
do not know what we do not know,
that is true knowledge.*

—NICOLAUS COPERNICUS

Women's Health

Baker, Jeannine Parvati. *Hygieia: A Woman's Herbal.* July 1986

Bennett, Jane, and Alexandra Pope. *The Pill: Are You Sure It's For You?* Allen and Unwin, Australia, 2008

Busteed, Marilyn, and Dorothy Wergin. *Phases of the Moon.* American Federation of Astrologers, Inc., AZ, 1992

Calais-German, Blandine. *The Female Pelvis: Anatomy & Exercises.* Eastland Press, Seattle, WA, 2003

Crawford, Amanda McQuade. *The Herbal Menopause Book.* The Crossing Press, 1999

Herbal Remedies for Women. Prima Publishing, 1997

Gladstar, Rosemary. *Herbal Healing for Women,* Simon & Schuster, New York, 1993

Herrera, Isa. *Ending Female Pain: A Woman's Manual.* Duplex Publishing, NY, 2009

Kent, Christine Ann. *Saving the Whole Woman.* Bridgeworks, NM, 2003

Kent, Tami Lynn. *Wild Feminine.* Tami Kent, MSPT, LLC, USA, 2008

Love, Susan M. *Dr. Susan Love's Hormone Book: Making Informed Choices about Menopause.* Times Books, Random House, NY, 1998

Northrup, Christiane. *The Wisdom of Menopause.* Bantam Books, 2003

Women's Bodies, Women's Wisdom. Bantam Books, 1994

Sarasohn, Lisa. *The Woman's Belly Book: Finding Your Treasure Within.* Self Health Education, Inc., North Carolina, 2003

Soule, Deb. *The Roots of Healing, A Woman's Book of Herbs.* Carol Publishing Group, 1995

Sperlich, Mickey. *Survivor Moms: Women's Stories of Birthing, Mothering and Healing after Sexual Abuse.* 2008

Trickey, Ruth. *Women, Hormones and the Menstrual Cycle: Herbal and Medical Solutions from Adolescence to Menopause.* Allen and Unwin, Australia, 2003

Weed, Susun. *The Menopausal Year.* Ashtree Publishing, NY, 1992

_____ and Alan McKnight. *Down There: Sexual and Reproductive Health the Wise Woman Way.* 2011

Weschler, Toni. *Cycle Savvy.* Collins, NY, 2006

Wiley, T.S. *Sex, Lies and Menopause: The Shocking Truth about Hormone Replacement Therapy.* Harper Collins, NY, 2003

Men's Health

Buhner, Stephen Harrod. *Vital Man, Natural Health Care for Men at Midlife.* Avery, NY, 2003

Green, James. *The Male Herbal, Health Care for Men and Boys.* The Crossing Press, CA, 1991

Herrera, Isa. *Ending Male Pelvic Pain: A Man's Manual.* Duplex Publishing, NY, 2013

Schultz, R. Louis. *Out in the Open, The Complete Male Pelvis.* North Atlantic Books, Berkeley, CA, 1999

Conception & Fertility

Baker, Jeannine Parvati, and Frederick Baker. *Conscious Conception.* Freestone Publishing Company, Utah and California, 1997

Indichova, Julia. *The Fertile Female: How the Power of Longing for a Child Can Save Your Life and Change the World.* Adell Press, 2007

Schwartz, James. *The Mind-Body Fertility Connection.* Llewellyn Publications, MN, 2008

Singer, Katie. *The Garden of Fertility.* Avery, NY, 2004

Weschler, Toni. *Taking Charge of Your Fertility,* 10th edition. Collins, 2006

Pregnancy and Childbirth

Gaskin, Ina May. *Spiritual Midwifery,* fourth edition. Book Publishing Company, TN, 2002

Ina May's Guide to Childbirth. Bantam Books, NY, 2003

Simkin, Penny, et al. *Pregnancy, Childbirth, and the Newborn: The Complete Guide,* 4th edition. Meadowbrook Press, Minnesota, 2010

Simkim, Penny, and Ruth Ancheta. *The Labor Progress Handbook: Early Interventions to Prevent and Treat Dystocia.* Wiley-Blackwell, 2011

Simkin, Penny and Phyllis Klaus. *When Survivors Give Birth: Understanding and Healing the Effects of Early Sexual Abuse on Childbearing Women.* 2004

England, Pam, and Rob Horowitz. *Birthing from Within: An Extra-Ordinary Guide to Childbirth.* Partera Press, NM, 1998

Kent, Tami Lynn, et al. *Mothering from Your Center: Tapping Your Body's Natural Energy for Pregnancy, Birth, and Parenting.* Atria Books/Beyond Words, 2013

Odent, Michel. *Childbirth and the Future of Homo Sapiens.* Printer & Martin, Great Britain, 2013

Digestive Health

Gershon, Michael. *The Second Brain: A Groundbreaking New Understanding of Nervous Disorders of the Stomach and Intestine.* HarperCollins, 1999

Mullin, Gerard E. *Integrative Gastroenterology.* Oxford University Press, 2011

General Reference

Eden, Donna. *Energy Medicine.* Jeremy P. Tarcher/Putnam, NY, 1998

Edelman, Hope. *The Possibility of Everything: A Memoir.* Ballantine Books, 2010

Judith, Anodea, and Selene Vega. *The Sevenfold Journey.* The Crossing Press, CA, 1993

Mate, Gabor. *When the Body Says No: Exploring the Stress-Disease Connection.* Alfred. A. Knopf, Canada, 2003

McGarey, William A. *The Oil That Heals,* 5th printing. ARE Press, VA, January 1999

Myss, Carolyn. *Anatomy of the Spirit: The Seven Stages of Power and Healing.* Crown Publishing, 1996

Pert, Candace. *Molecules of Emotion: The Science behind Mind-Body Medicine.* Touchstone. 1999

Rector-Page, Linda. *Healthy Healing: An Alternative Reference.* Healthy Healing Publications. 1992

Weed, Susun S. *Healing Wise.* Ash Tree Publishing, NY, 1989

Books by Dr. Arvigo

Arvigo, Rosita. *Food of the Gods: A Vegetarian Cookbook from Belize* (self published)

Medicinal Plants Used in Northern Guanajuato

_____ and Michael Balick. *Rainforest Remedies: 100 Healing Herbs from Belize.* Lotus Press, 1993

_____ and Nadine Epstein. *Sastun, My Apprenticeship with a Maya Shaman.* Harper Collins, 1997

_____ and Nadine Epstein. *101 Rainforest Home Remedies.* Harper Collins, 2001

_____ and Nadine Epstein. *Spiritual Bathing Traditions from Around the World.* Ten Speed Press, 2003

Condition References

Assisted Reproductive Technology

"Infertility FAQs," Division of Reproductive Health, National Center for Chronic Disease Prevention and Health Promotion, Centers for Disease Control and Prevention, June 2013 http://www.cdc.gov/reproductivehealth/Infertility/index.htm

"IVF Babies Have Greater Risk of Complications, Study Finds," Ian Sample, the *Guardian,* January 8, 2014 http://www.theguardian.com/society/2014/jan/08/ivf-babies-risk-complications-study

Benign Prostatic Hyperplasia

"Benign Prostatic Hyperplasia (BPH, Enlarged Prostate)," Glenn Gerber, MD, MedicineNet, December 2013 http://www.medicinenet.com/benign_prostatic_hyperplasia/article.htm

Chronic Constipation

"Chronic Constipation," Center for Neurobiology of Stress, UCLA http://uclacns.org/patients/disease-information/chronic-constipation/

"Constipation," National Digestive Diseases Information Clearinghouse, National Institute of Diabetes and Digestive and Kidney Diseases, National Institutes of Health http://digestive.niddk.nih.gov/ddiseases/pubs/constipation/

Colitis

"Colitis," Benjamin Wedro, MD, MedicineNet, August 2013 http://www.medicinenet.com/colitis/article.htm

Dysmenorrhea

"Dysmenorrhea," FAQ 046, American College of Obstetricians and Gynecologists, July 2012 http://www.acog.org/~/media/For%20 Patients/faq046.pdf?dmc=1&ts=20140211T1659579272

"Primary dysmenorrhea and uterine blood flow: a color Doppler study," S. Altunyurt et al., *Journal of Reproductive Medicine,* April 2005 http://www.ncbi.nlm.nih.gov/pubmed/15916208

Endometriosis

"Endometriosis," FAQ 013, American College of Obstetricians and Gynecologists, October 2012 http://www.acog.org/~/media/For%20 Patients/faq013.pdf?dmc=1&ts=20140211T1732493530

Fibroids

"Fibroids," FAQ 074, American College of Obstetricians and Gynecologists, May 2011 http://www.acog.org/~/media/For%20Patients/faq074. pdf?dmc=1&ts=20140215T0758566767

"Uterine Fibroids (Benign Tumors of the Uterus)," Melissa Conrad Stöppler, MD, MedicineNet, January 2014 http://www.medicinenet.com/ uterine_fibroids/article.htm

Gastroparesis

"Gastroparesis," Jay W. Marks, MD, MedicineNet, June 2012 http://www. medicinenet.com/gastroparesis/article.htm

"Gastroparesis: Concepts, Controversies, and Challenges," Klaus Bielefeldt, *Scientifica,* July 2012 http://www.hindawi.com/journals/ scientifica/2012/424802/

Infant Acid Reflux

"Ask Dr. Sears: Coping with Baby's Acid Reflux," Dr. William Sears, *Parenting,* 2011 http://www.parenting.com/article/ask-dr-sears-coping-with-babys-acid-reflux

Infertility

"Infertility," reviewed by Susan Storck, MD, A.D.A.M. Medical Encyclopedia, PubMed Health, February 2013 http://www.ncbi.nlm.nih.gov/pubmedhealth/PMH0002173/

"Infertility FAQs," Division of Reproductive Health, National Center for Chronic Disease Prevention and Health Promotion, Centers for Disease Control and Prevention, June 2013 http://www.cdc.gov/reproductivehealth/Infertility/index.htm

"What Is Infertility?," Resolve: The National Infertility Association http://www.resolve.org/infertility-overview/what-is-infertility/

Irritable Bowel Syndrome

"About Irritable Bowel Syndrome (IBS)," International Foundation for Functional Gastrointestinal Disorders, February 2014 http://www.aboutibs.org/

"Irritable Bowel Syndrome," reviewed by David C. Dugdale, III, MD, A.D.A.M. Medical Encyclopedia, PubMed Health, July 2011 http://www.ncbi.nlm.nih.gov/pubmedhealth/PMH0001292/

Polycystic Ovary Syndrome

"Polycystic Ovary Syndrome," FAQ 121, American College of Obstetricians and Gynecologists, August 2011 http://www.acog.org/~/media/For%20Patients/faq121.pdf?dmc=1&ts=20140212T1247248413

"Polycystic Ovary Syndrome (PCOS)—Topic Overview," Women's Health, WebMD, February 2012 http://www.webmd.com/women/tc/polycystic-ovary-syndrome-pcos-topic-overview

Pelvic Organ Prolapse

"Female Urology—Vaginal or Pelvic Organ Prolapse (POP)," Columbia Urology, Columbia University Medical Center http://columbiaurology.org/specialties/female/vaginal-prolapse.html

"Pelvic Support Problems," FAQ 012, American College of Obstetricians and Gynecologists, May 2011 http://www.acog.org/~/media/For%20Patients/faq012.pdf?dmc=1&ts=20140211T2127041264

Prostatitis/Chronic Pelvic Pain Syndrome

"Chronic Prostatitis and Chronic Pelvic Pain in Men: Aetiology, Diagnosis and Management," G. A. Luzzi, *Journal of the European Academy of Dermatology and Venereology,* May 2002 http://www.ncbi.nlm.nih.gov/pubmed/12195565

"Epidemiology and Evaluation of Chronic Pelvic Pain Syndrome in Men," A. J. Schaeffer, *International Journal of Antimicrobial Agents,* February 2008 http://www.ncbi.nlm.nih.gov/pubmed/18164597

Secondary Infertility

"Subsequent Obstetric Performance Related to Primary Mode of Delivery," J. Jolly et al., *British Journal of Obstetrics and Gynaecology* [now called *BJOG: An International Journal of Obstetrics and Gynaecology*], March 1999 http://www.ncbi.nlm.nih.gov/pubmed/?term=subsequent+obstetric+performance+related+to+primary+mode+of+delivery

"What Is Secondary Infertility?," PreconceptionWeekly, ParentingWeekly http://www.parentingweekly.com/preconception/preconception_information/secondary_infertility.htm

Sexual Trauma (Practitioner Note, M. Sperlich)

"Childhood Sexual Abuse and Adult Psychiatric Substance Use Disorders in Women," K. S. Kendler et al., *Archives of General Psychiatry,* October 2000 http://www.ncbi.nlm.nih.gov/pubmed/11015813

"Examining the Unique Relationships between Anxiety Disorders and Childhood Physical and Sexual Abuse in the National Comorbidity Survey-Replication," J. R. Cougle et al., *Psychiatry Research,* May 2010 http://www.ncbi.nlm.nih.gov/pubmed/20381878

"A Global Perspective on Child Sexual Abuse: Meta-analysis of Prevalence around the World," by M. Stoltenborgh et al., *Child Maltreatment,* May 2011 http://www.ncbi.nlm.nih.gov/pubmed/21511741

"The International Epidemiology of Child Sexual Abuse: A Continuation of Finkelhor (1994)," N. Pereda et al., *Child Abuse & Neglect,* June 2009 http://www.ncbi.nlm.nih.gov/pubmed/19477003

"Prevalence and Psychological Sequelae of Self-Reported Childhood Physical and Sexual Abuse in a General Sample of Men and Women," J. Briere et al., *Child Abuse & Neglect,* October 2003 http://www.ncbi.nlm.nih.gov/pubmed/14602100

"The Prevalence of Child Sexual Abuse: Integrative Review Adjustment for Potential Response Bias and Measurement Biases," K. M. Gorey et al., *Child Abuse & Neglect,* April 1997 http://www.ncbi.nlm.nih.gov/pubmed/9134267

Urinary Tract Infection

"What I Need to Know about Urinary Tract Infections," National Kidney and Urologic Diseases Information Clearinghouse, National Institute of Diabetes and Digestive and Kidney Diseases, National Institutes of Health, September 2013 http://kidney.niddk.nih.gov/kudiseases/pubs/uti_ez/#1

Vaginal Birth after Caesarean (VBAC)

"Births—Method of Delivery," FastStats, National Center for Health Statistics, Centers for Disease Control and Prevention, 2012 http://www.cdc.gov/nchs/fastats/delivery.htm

"Making Informed Decisions about VBAC or Repeat Cesareans," January 2014 http://www.vbac.com/making-informed-decisions-about-vbac-or-repeat-cesareans/

"Vaginal Birth after Cesarean FAQ," Childbirth.org http://www.childbirth.org/section/VBACFAQ.html

Index of Conditions